The Perricone Weight-Loss Diet Personal Journal

The Perricone Weight-Loss Diet Personal Journal

A Simple 3-Part Plan to Lose the Fat, the Wrinkles, and the Years

Nicholas Perricone, M.D.

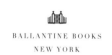

BALLANTINE BOOKS
NEW YORK

No book can replace the diagnostic expertise and medical advice of a trusted physician. Please be certain to consult with your doctor before making any decisions that affect your health, particularly if you suffer from any medical condition or have any symptom that may require treatment.

A Ballantine Books Trade Paperback Original

Copyright © 2006 by Nicholas V. Perricone, M.D.

Published in the United States by Ballantine Books, an imprint of The Random House Publishing Group, a division of Random House, Inc., New York.

BALLANTINE and colophon are registered trademarks of Random House, Inc.

ISBN 0-345-49133-5

Printed in the United States of America

www.ballantinebooks.com

987654321

Book design by Eli Brown

The Perricone Weight-Loss Diet
Personal Daily Journal

Of

_____

Introduction

Welcome and thank you for choosing *The Perricone Weight-Loss Diet* to reach your weight-loss goals. I am delighted to present here important tools that have been proven to work—every time.

Many of my patients and readers were surprised when they heard that I was writing a book on weight loss. However, once you understand what is at the basis of unwanted weight gain and obesity, it will make perfect sense.

My two decades as a dermatologist and anti-aging expert have taught me one very important concept: *invisible, sub-clinical inflammation is the final common pathway in a wide variety of diseases and degenerative conditions including heart disease, certain forms of cancer, Alzheimer's disease, diabetes, metabolic syndrome, acne, many of the signs of aging, and excess weight.*

My early research indicated that food had a tremendous influence on this inflammation and, depending on the foods and beverages we chose, could either increase or decrease inflammation in the body. This led me to develop what I call the anti-inflammatory diet, the foundation for an internal approach to staying young and living a longer, healthier life. The way to accomplish this is by decreasing the micro-inflammation that goes on in our cells all day, every day.

As I continued to introduce thousands of patients to the anti-inflammatory diet over the years, I quickly discovered that those patients who had extra body fat rapidly lost weight. I continued to perfect the program, adding lifestyle modifications and key nutritional supplements to facilitate weight loss while maintaining muscle mass. The good news was that not one of the people who lost weight on this plan looked haggard or tired—symptoms many report when they embark on a weight-loss regimen.

In this journal you will find an easy-to-follow daily meal plan, the ideal foods to mix and match from all food groups, and many important tips to speed you to your goals—long-term, safe, permanent weight loss.

In addition, you will find that the benefits are not just in the area of weight loss. Your skin will take on a new youthfulness and radiance, your mind and memory will be sharp and your mood elevated.

The foods and beverages on the Perricone Weight-Loss Diet will also increase your energy and your ability to sleep, and will enhance your sense of well-being.

I have learned that my patients who keep a journal achieve the greatest success. Keeping a written report is a great motivator and will keep you focused on your goals.

The journal will help you to chronicle each exciting, life-changing day and bear written testament to your remarkable transformation.

I wish you success and joy as you embark on this journey and trust that the Perricone Weight-Loss Diet will improve the quality of your life for many years to come.

Nicholas Perricone, M.D.
Madison, Connecticut

DAY 1

"BEFORE" PHOTO

TOTAL BODY WEIGHT: _____

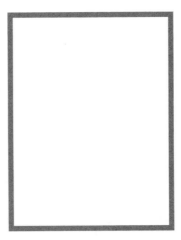

DAY 28

"AFTER" PHOTO

TOTAL BODY WEIGHT: _____

Getting Started

STEP 1: THE FOODS

As a basic guideline, here is a list of the recommended foods for The Perricone Weight-Loss Diet.

At the back of this journal is a Resources section telling you where to get some of the recommended selections on this page. Please see *The Perricone Weight-Loss Diet* for more information on the Top 10 Food Groups for Permanent Weight Loss as well as for all recipes listed in the daily meal plans.

OMEGA-3 SEAFOOD

- Anchovies
- Bass
- Halibut
- Herring
- Mackerel
- Sablefish
- Sardines
- Trout
- Wild Alaskan salmon—Sockeye salmon has the highest amount of omega-3 of any fish: about 2.7 grams per 100 gram portion.

ADDITIONAL SEAFOOD RECOMMENDATIONS

- Clams
- Cod
- Crab
- Flounder
- Lobster
- Mussels
- Oysters
- Scallops
- Shrimp

BEST POULTRY CHOICES

- Cornish hens
- Organic, free range chicken and turkey
- Turkey sausage and bacon (avoid any products with nitrates, also called nitrites)

BEST SOURCES OF PROTEIN FROM DAIRY

- Plain kefir
- Plain low-fat organic yogurt
- Organic eggs from free range, cage-free chickens, labeled "Omega-3"
- Organic low-fat cottage cheese

ORGANIC, UNSALTED NUTS AND SEEDS

- Almonds
- Brazil nuts
- Hazelnuts (filberts)
- Macadamia
- Pecans
- Pine nuts (pignoli nuts)
- Pistachios
- Walnuts

ORGANIC UNSALTED SEEDS

- Flaxseed
- Pumpkin and squash seeds
- Sesame seeds
- Sunflower seeds

ORGANIC GRAINS AND LEGUMES— USE IN MODERATION FOR WEIGHT LOSS

- Barley
- Buckwheat
- Chickpeas
- Dried beans
- Lentils
- Old-fashioned non-instant oatmeal or whole oats

FRUITS AND VEGETABLES

- Apples
- Arugula
- Artichokes
- Asparagus
- Avocado
- Blueberries, blackberries, strawberries, raspberries (all berries)
- Bamboo shoots
- Bok choy
- Broccoli
- Broccoli rabe
- Brussels sprouts
- Cabbage
- Cauliflower
- Cantaloupe
- Celery
- Cherries
- Chicory
- Chinese cabbage
- Collards
- Cucumbers
- Dark green leafy lettuces (baby greens)
- Eggplant
- Endive
- Escarole
- Fresh lemons
- Grapefruit
- Greens (turnip, collard, mustard, dark lettuce)
- Green beans
- Green and red bell peppers
- Honeydew melon

- Hot peppers
- Jerusalem artichokes
- Kale
- Mushrooms
- Onions, garlic, chives, leeks, scallions, etc.
- Pears
- Pea pods
- Radishes
- Rutabaga
- Swiss chard
- Spinach
- Sprouts of all kinds
- Summer squash
- Tomatoes
- Turnips
- Water chestnuts
- Zucchini

HERBS AND SPICES

- Anise
- Allspice
- Basil
- Bay leaf
- Caraway
- Cardamom
- Cayenne
- Celery seed
- Chili flakes
- Chives
- Chervil
- Cilantro
- Cinnamon
- Clove
- Coriander
- Cumin
- Dill
- Fennel
- Garlic
- Ginger
- Lemon balm
- Mace
- Marjoram
- Mint
- Nutmeg
- Oregano
- Paprika (sweet and hot)
- Parsley
- Peppercorns (black, green, white, pink)
- Rosemary
- Sage
- Saffron
- Savory
- Tarragon
- Turmeric
- Thyme
- Vanilla bean

BEVERAGES

- Açaí (found in natural food stores)
- Cocoa (made with pure cocoa powder and Stevia)
- Jana Skinny Water™
- Organic black tea
- Organic green tea
- Organic white tea
- Pomegranate juice (unsweetened)
- Water (pure spring water like Fiji or Poland Spring)

SWEETENERS

- Agave
- Stevia (available at health food stores and some markets)

HEALTHY FATS

- Avocado
- Chocolate (as described in text)
- Coconut/coconut oil
- Flax oil
- Nuts and seeds
- Olives
- Organic extra virgin olive oil (look for Italian or Spanish high quality)

STEP 2: THE NUTRITIONAL SUPPLEMENTS

It is important that you consult with your primary physician before embarking on a new supplement program—this is absolutely vital if you are taking any medications or are being treated for any medical condition.

You may take the recommended supplements listed below in addition to your regular multivitamin. Please consult *The Perricone Weight-Loss Diet* for dosage recommendations. I have also created Weight Management Supplements. These are already pre-packaged in individual packets for your convenience. Take one packet with each meal (for a total of 3 packets per day) along with three omega-3 fish oil capsules and ½ teaspoon of glutamine powder. Note: check the Resources section for sources of these packets and individual supplements.

Always take your pills with a full glass of water (at least eight ounces).

RECOMMENDED SUPPLEMENTS FOR THE PERRICONE WEIGHT-LOSS DIET

- Omega-3 Fish Oil
- Alpha Lipoic Acid (ALA)
- Astaxanthin
- Carnitine
- Acetyl-L-carnitine
- Conjugated Linoleic Acid (CLA)
- Coenzyme Q10 (CoQ10)
- Chromium
- Glutamine
- Gamma Linolenic Acid (GLA)
- Maitake SX-fraction™
- Dimethylaminoethanol (DMAE)

STEP 3: THE ANTI-INFLAMMATORY LIFESTYLE

Food isn't the only thing that makes us fat. An amazingly large number of factors, from how much sleep we get to how much water we drink, can trigger or inhibit the inflammatory response. To maximize the weight loss and health benefits of eating anti-inflammatory foods and taking the supplements recommended above, be sure to make time for regular, moderate exercise and stress reduction:

- ◆   Establish a regular exercise plan
- ◆   Make time for quiet contemplation
- ◆   Follow a basic routine
- ◆   Get enough sleep
- ◆   Drink enough water
- ◆   Spend time with people and pets you love

STEP 4: THE JOURNAL

The next section of the book contains the actual daily plan and the journal part. Follow the many tips and record your progress on a daily basis. You are embarking on a way of living that will not only help you lose weight and keep your weight down, it will also make you healthier and happier for the rest of your life. The left page will have that day's meal plan. You don't have to be a slave to it. Be creative. As long as you choose foods from the recommended list, feel free to mix and match—just make sure that you include protein, low-glycemic carbs such as antioxidant-rich fruits and veggies, and essential fats with each meal and snack. All recipes can be found in *The Perricone Weight-Loss Diet*, available in hardcover from Ballantine Books.

When you begin the journal, it is important to fill out the positive benefits you are feeling because they are a great motivator. Even if you are just starting and have no weight loss to report, writing down the positives is still necessary—just starting the program is a reward in and of itself.

If you felt tired or depressed, had a double latte and croissant and got zero exercise for the day, that's okay, too. Record it all—when you are tempted to fall into bad habits the journal will give you renewed focus.

You will look and feel different in as little as three days. The goal of this journal is to help you record the physical, mental, emotional, and spiritual benefits you will experience, to keep you healthy, happy, and motivated.

Don't be mystified by the "three things to celebrate" category. It can be as uplifting and simple as hugging your cat or dog, enjoying a walk on a beautiful day, or feeling the satisfaction of taking proactive steps toward improving the quality of your life.

An added benefit of The Perricone Weight-Loss Diet is that your skin will glow with a new youthfulness—that look of health, vitality and radiance you may have thought was lost forever.

Always remember to eat the protein first at every meal.

WEEK 1 / DAY 1   DATE: _____

BREAKFAST:

- 2 poached omega-3 eggs with **Indian Spinach***
- 2 slices turkey bacon
- ½ cup honeydew with 1 teaspoon chopped fresh mint
- 8 ounces green tea with slice of ginger or spring water

Supplements:

- 1 packet of Weight Management supplements
- 1 1,000 mg fish oil capsule
- 1 astaxanthin capsule
- ½ teaspoon glutamine powder—mix in water and drink immediately

LUNCH:

- 1½ cups **African Groundnut Stew***
- 1 cup of salad (dark green leafy lettuce, dressed with 1 tablespoon extra virgin olive oil; fresh lemon juice to taste)
- ⅓ cup berries
- 8 ounces spring water

Supplements:

- 1 packet of Weight Management supplements
- 1 1,000 mg fish oil capsule
- 1 astaxanthin capsule
- ½ teaspoon glutamine powder—mix in water and drink immediately

* All recipes can be found in *The Perricone Weight-Loss Diet*

> Animal fats are pro-inflammatory saturated fats, so use them in moderation.

SNACK:

- ¼ cup **Edamame Guacamole*** + 1 teaspoon flaxseed served with celery and jicama sticks
- 8 ounces spring water

DINNER:

- Poached or grilled salmon (6–8 ounces raw weight) with **Spring Roll Salad***
- Steamed asparagus
- 2-inch wedge of cantaloupe
- 8 ounces spring water

Supplements:

- 1 packet of Weight Management supplements
- 1 1,000 mg fish oil capsule
- 1 astaxanthin capsule
- ½ teaspoon glutamine powder—mix in water and drink immediately

BEDTIME:

- ¼ cup plain yogurt with ½ teaspoon vanilla
- 1 teaspoon ground flax
- ¼ cup raspberries
- **Moroccan Mint Tea*** or spring water

* All recipes can be found in *The Perricone Weight-Loss Diet*

JOURNAL NOTES

THREE THINGS TO CELEBRATE FROM MY DAY:

1. _____

2. _____

3. _____

RECORD THE POSITIVE CHANGES
YOUR BODY EXPERIENCES EACH DAY

Weight: _____   Tone: _____

Energy: _____

Exercise: _____

RECORD THE POSITIVE MENTAL AND
EMOTIONAL EXPERIENCES EACH DAY

Changes in mood: _____

Stress handling: _____

Memory: _____

Problem-solving ability: _____

EMBRACING THE ANTI-INFLAMMATORY LIFESTYLE

Progress in overcoming bad habits:

_____

Progress in minimizing stress:

_____

Cups of coffee: _____   Alcohol: _____

Smoking: _____   Conflict/Tension: _____

Sleep (# of hours): _____   Sleep quality: _____

BENEFITS OF THE GIFT OF QUIET CONTEMPLATION

_____

_____

_____

_____

_____

_____

_____

_____

_____

> Every meal or snack must include protein, low-glycemic carbs, and essential fatty acids.

WEEK 1 / DAY 2　　　　　　　　DATE: _____

BREAKFAST:

◆ 2 soft-boiled eggs

◆ ½ cup (measured dry) **Stop the Clock! Cereal*** with 1 tablespoon POM Wonderful pomegranate juice or pure açaí pulp

◆ ½ cup plain yogurt with ½ cup diced cantaloupe and 1 teaspoon chopped mint

◆ 8 ounces green tea or spring water

Supplements:

◆ 1 packet of Weight Management supplements

◆ 1 1,000 mg fish oil capsule

◆ 1 astaxanthin capsule

◆ ½ teaspoon glutamine powder—mix in water and drink immediately

LUNCH:

◆ **Icy Gazpacho with Fresh Lime***

◆ Grilled chicken breast (6 ounces raw weight boneless skinless)

◆ 1 cup of salad (dark green leafy lettuce, dressed with 1 tablespoon extra virgin olive oil; fresh lemon juice to taste)

◆ ½ grapefruit

◆ 8 ounces iced green tea or spring water

Supplements:

◆ 1 packet of Weight Management supplements

◆ 1 1,000 mg fish oil capsule

◆ 1 astaxanthin capsule

◆ ½ teaspoon glutamine powder—mix in water and drink immediately

* All recipes can be found in *The Perricone Weight-Loss Diet*

> **Omega-3 fatty acids found in fish and fish oil help us burn off calories before they get a chance to be stored as fat.**

SNACK:

♦ ⅓ cup cottage cheese with 1 tablespoon ground flax and ¼ cup blueberries

♦ 8 ounces spring water

DINNER:

♦ Poached or baked halibut (or salmon) (6–8 ounces raw weight boneless) with **Curried Cabbage***

♦ 1 cup of cherry tomato salad with 1 teaspoon each chopped ginger, cilantro, extra virgin olive oil; low-sodium soy sauce and fresh lemon juice to taste

♦ 1 pear

♦ 8 ounces spring water with fresh lime

Supplements:

♦ 1 packet of Weight Management supplements

♦ 1 1,000 mg fish oil capsule

♦ 1 astaxanthin capsule

♦ ½ teaspoon glutamine powder—mix in water and drink immediately

BEDTIME:

♦ ½ cup kefir

♦ 3 almonds

♦ 6 cherries

♦ 8 ounces spring water

* All recipes can be found in *The Perricone Weight-Loss Diet*

JOURNAL NOTES

THREE THINGS TO CELEBRATE FROM MY DAY:

1. _____

2. _____

3. _____

RECORD THE POSITIVE CHANGES
YOUR BODY EXPERIENCES EACH DAY

Weight: _____   Tone: _____

Energy: _____

Exercise: _____

RECORD THE POSITIVE MENTAL AND
EMOTIONAL EXPERIENCES EACH DAY

Changes in mood: _____

Stress handling: _____

Memory: _____

Problem-solving ability: _____

EMBRACING THE ANTI-INFLAMMATORY LIFESTYLE

Progress in overcoming bad habits:

_____

Progress in minimizing stress:

_____

Cups of coffee: _____   Alcohol: _____

Smoking: _____   Conflict/Tension: _____

Sleep (# of hours): _____   Sleep quality: _____

BENEFITS OF THE GIFT OF QUIET CONTEMPLATION

_____

_____

_____

_____

_____

_____

_____

_____

_____

> **Always eat your protein first.**
> **This will help suppress your appetite.**

WEEK 1 / DAY 3   DATE: _____

BREAKFAST:

♦ 2 whole eggs plus two egg whites scrambled with 1 slice turkey bacon and **Nutty Tomato Pesto***

♦ ½ grapefruit

♦ 8 ounces green tea or spring water

Supplements:

♦ 1 packet of Weight Management supplements

♦ 1 1,000 mg fish oil capsule

♦ 1 astaxanthin capsule

♦ ½ teaspoon glutamine powder—mix in water and drink immediately

LUNCH:

♦ Salmon fillet, baked or grilled (4–6 ounces raw weight boneless) with 1 cup **Caponata*** salad served on mixed baby greens

♦ ½ cup raspberries

♦ 8 ounces iced white or green tea or spring water

Supplements:

♦ 1 packet of Weight Management supplements

♦ 1 1,000 mg fish oil capsule

♦ 1 astaxanthin capsule

♦ ½ teaspoon glutamine powder—mix in water and drink immediately

* All recipes can be found in *The Perricone Weight-Loss Diet*

> A good night's sleep can help you wake
> refreshed, looking radiant and youthful.
> And, after a good night's sleep, doesn't the
> world look better, too?

SNACK:

◆ Smoothie with ½ cup kefir, 1 teaspoon ground flax, and ½ cup sliced strawberries

◆ 8 ounces spring water

DINNER:

◆ Grilled shrimp (6 ounces raw weight)

◆ **Scalloped Tomatoes with Caramelized Onions***

◆ 1 cup of salad (dark green leafy lettuce, dressed with 1 tablespoon extra virgin olive oil; fresh lemon juice to taste)

◆ 1 apple

◆ 8 ounces spring water

Supplements:

◆ 1 packet of Weight Management supplements

◆ 1 1,000 mg fish oil capsule

◆ 1 astaxanthin capsule

◆ ½ teaspoon glutamine powder—mix in water and drink immediately

BEDTIME:

◆ 1 ounce sliced smoked salmon with 2 flax crackers

◆ 1 kiwi

◆ 8 ounces spring water

* All recipes can be found in *The Perricone Weight-Loss Diet*

JOURNAL NOTES

THREE THINGS TO CELEBRATE FROM MY DAY:

1. _____

2. _____

3. _____

RECORD THE POSITIVE CHANGES
YOUR BODY EXPERIENCES EACH DAY

Weight: _____   Tone: _____

Energy: _____

Exercise: _____

RECORD THE POSITIVE MENTAL AND
EMOTIONAL EXPERIENCES EACH DAY

Changes in mood: _____

Stress handling: _____

Memory: _____

Problem-solving ability: _____

EMBRACING THE ANTI-INFLAMMATORY LIFESTYLE

Progress in overcoming bad habits:

_____

Progress in minimizing stress:

_____

Cups of coffee: _____   Alcohol: _____

Smoking: _____   Conflict/Tension: _____

Sleep (# of hours): _____   Sleep quality: _____

BENEFITS OF THE GIFT OF QUIET CONTEMPLATION

_____

_____

_____

_____

_____

_____

_____

_____

_____

Save the fresh fruit for the end of the meal. This will prevent the natural sugars found in the fruit from causing a spike in blood sugar.

WEEK 1 / DAY 4   DATE: _____

BREAKFAST:

- 1 boiled egg
- ½ cup **Stop the Clock! Cereal***
- ½ cup **Blueberry Compote*** with 1 cup plain yogurt
- 8 ounces green or white tea or spring water

Supplements:

- 1 packet of Weight Management supplements
- 1 1,000 mg fish oil capsule
- 1 astaxanthin capsule
- ½ teaspoon glutamine powder—mix in water and drink immediately

LUNCH:

- Grilled turkey burger (4–6 ounces raw weight) served on baby spinach
- Tossed green salad with ¼ avocado slice
- 1 apple
- 8 ounces iced green tea with lemon or spring water

Supplements:

- 1 packet of Weight Management supplements
- 1 1,000 mg fish oil capsule
- 1 astaxanthin capsule
- ½ teaspoon glutamine powder—mix in water and drink immediately

* All recipes can be found in *The Perricone Weight-Loss Diet*

> Essential fatty acids found in fish and fish oil lower insulin levels. High levels of insulin cause weight gain and block weight loss.

SNACK:

♦ Cantaloupe wedge wrapped with 1 ounce slice of turkey breast, drizzled with 1 teaspoon flax oil

♦ 8 ounces spring water

DINNER:

♦ Grilled salmon (6–8 ounces raw weight) with **Creamy Onion Sauce with Roasted Garlic and Thyme***

♦ Steamed artichoke

♦ 1 cup of salad (dark green leafy lettuce, dressed with 1 tablespoon extra virgin olive oil; fresh lemon juice to taste)

♦ 8 ounces spring water

Supplements:

♦ 1 packet of Weight Management supplements

♦ 1 1,000 mg fish oil capsule

♦ 1 astaxanthin capsule

♦ ½ teaspoon glutamine powder—mix in water and drink immediately

BEDTIME:

♦ ¼ cup yogurt mixed with 1 tablespoon POM Wonderful pomegranate juice or pure açaí pulp

♦ 2 tablespoons sliced almonds

♦ ½ kiwi, diced

♦ 8 ounces spring water

* All recipes can be found in *The Perricone Weight-Loss Diet*

JOURNAL NOTES

THREE THINGS TO CELEBRATE FROM MY DAY:

1. _____

2. _____

3. _____

RECORD THE POSITIVE CHANGES
YOUR BODY EXPERIENCES EACH DAY

Weight: _____   Tone: _____

Energy: _____

Exercise: _____

RECORD THE POSITIVE MENTAL AND
EMOTIONAL EXPERIENCES EACH DAY

Changes in mood: _____

Stress handling: _____

Memory: _____

Problem-solving ability: _____

EMBRACING THE ANTI-INFLAMMATORY LIFESTYLE

Progress in overcoming bad habits:

_____

Progress in minimizing stress:

_____

Cups of coffee: _____   Alcohol: _____

Smoking: _____   Conflict/Tension: _____

Sleep (# of hours): _____   Sleep quality: _____

BENEFITS OF THE GIFT OF QUIET CONTEMPLATION

_____

_____

_____

_____

_____

_____

_____

_____

> Looking for a fat-burner, muscle-builder, wrinkle-eraser, skin-saver, depression-lifter, and brain-booster? Try wild Alaskan salmon!

WEEK 1 / DAY 5   DATE: _____

BREAKFAST:

◆ 2 egg omelet with 2 ounces smoked salmon, fresh dill, and cherry tomatoes

◆ ⅓ cup kefir with 2 tablespoons blackberries

◆ 8 ounces green or white tea or spring water

Supplements:

◆ 1 packet of Weight Management supplements

◆ 1 1,000 mg fish oil capsule

◆ 1 astaxanthin capsule

◆ ½ teaspoon glutamine powder—mix in water and drink immediately

LUNCH:

◆ 6 ounces **Egyptian Chicken Salad***

◆ 1 cup **Broccoli Dill Soup with Lemon and Tahini***

◆ 1 apple

◆ 8 ounces spring water

Supplements:

◆ 1 packet of Weight Management supplements

◆ 1 1,000 mg fish oil capsule

◆ 1 astaxanthin capsule

◆ ½ teaspoon glutamine powder—mix in water and drink immediately

* All recipes can be found in *The Perricone Weight-Loss Diet*

> Our goal is to avoid spikes in blood sugar
> because they trigger insulin release.
> Remember this fact: insulin release = stored fat!

SNACK:

♦ ½ cup yogurt with 1 tablespoon chopped hazelnuts and ¼ cup diced kiwi

♦ 8 ounces spring water

DINNER:

♦ Grilled sablefish (or salmon) (6–8 ounces raw weight skinless)

♦ **Cucumber-Tomato Salad***

♦ **Brussels Sprouts with Slivered Almonds***

♦ 8 ounces spring water

Supplements:

♦ 1 packet of Weight Management supplements

♦ 1 1,000 mg fish oil capsule

♦ 1 astaxanthin capsule

♦ ½ teaspoon glutamine powder—mix in water and drink immediately

BEDTIME:

♦ ½ cup cottage cheese with 1 teaspoon ground flaxseed and ⅓ cup sliced strawberries

♦ 8 ounces spring water

* All recipes can be found in *The Perricone Weight-Loss Diet*

JOURNAL NOTES

THREE THINGS TO CELEBRATE FROM MY DAY:

1. _____

2. _____

3. _____

RECORD THE POSITIVE CHANGES
YOUR BODY EXPERIENCES EACH DAY

Weight: _____   Tone: _____

Energy: _____

Exercise: _____

RECORD THE POSITIVE MENTAL AND
EMOTIONAL EXPERIENCES EACH DAY

Changes in mood: _____

Stress handling: _____

Memory: _____

Problem-solving ability: _____

EMBRACING THE ANTI-INFLAMMATORY LIFESTYLE

Progress in overcoming bad habits:

_____

Progress in minimizing stress:

_____

Cups of coffee: _____   Alcohol: _____

Smoking: _____   Conflict/Tension: _____

Sleep (# of hours): _____   Sleep quality: _____

BENEFITS OF THE GIFT OF QUIET CONTEMPLATION

_____

_____

_____

_____

_____

_____

_____

_____

_____

> **If you don't drink water,
> your body cannot metabolize fat.**

WEEK 1 / DAY 6   DATE: _____

BREAKFAST:

- 2 hard-boiled omega-3 eggs
- ½ cup (measured dry) **Stop the Clock! Cereal***
- ⅓ cup blueberries or blackberries plus ¼ cup plain yogurt
- 8 ounces green tea with lemon or spring water

Supplements:

- 1 packet of Weight Management supplements
- 1 1,000 mg fish oil capsule
- 1 astaxanthin capsule
- ½ teaspoon glutamine powder—mix in water and drink immediately

LUNCH:

- Poached or baked salmon (4–6 ounces raw weight boneless)
- 1 cup **Persian Vegetable Soup***
- 1 2-inch wedge honeydew
- 8 ounces spring water

Supplements:

- 1 packet of Weight Management supplements
- 1 1,000 mg fish oil capsule
- 1 astaxanthin capsule
- ½ teaspoon glutamine powder—mix in water and drink immediately

* All recipes can be found in *The Perricone Weight-Loss Diet*

> Eat raw foods for enzymes. Enzymes are critical to good health as they assist in the digestion and absorption of nutrients from food.

SNACK:

♦ Smoothie with ½ cup kefir, 1 teaspoon flax oil, pinch of cinnamon, and 2 tablespoons raspberries

♦ 8 ounces spring water

DINNER:

♦ **Grilled Miso Salmon (or Chicken)*** (6–8 ounces raw weight)

♦ Sautéed spinach (or escarole) and mushrooms

♦ 1 cup of salad (dark green leafy lettuce, dressed with 1 tablespoon extra virgin olive oil; fresh lemon juice to taste)

♦ 1 apple

♦ 8 ounces green tea or spring water

Supplements:

♦ 1 packet of Weight Management supplements

♦ 1 1,000 mg fish oil capsule

♦ 1 astaxanthin capsule

♦ ½ teaspoon glutamine powder—mix in water and drink immediately

BEDTIME:

♦ 1 ounce slice smoked chicken

♦ 4 walnuts

♦ 1 2-inch wedge honeydew

♦ 8 ounces spring water

* All recipes can be found in *The Perricone Weight-Loss Diet*

JOURNAL NOTES

THREE THINGS TO CELEBRATE FROM MY DAY:

1. _____

2. _____

3. _____

RECORD THE POSITIVE CHANGES
YOUR BODY EXPERIENCES EACH DAY

Weight: _____   Tone: _____

Energy: _____

Exercise: _____

RECORD THE POSITIVE MENTAL AND
EMOTIONAL EXPERIENCES EACH DAY

Changes in mood: _____

Stress handling: _____

Memory: _____

Problem-solving ability: _____

EMBRACING THE ANTI-INFLAMMATORY LIFESTYLE

Progress in overcoming bad habits:

_____

Progress in minimizing stress:

_____

Cups of coffee: _____   Alcohol: _____

Smoking: _____   Conflict/Tension: _____

Sleep (# of hours): _____   Sleep quality: _____

BENEFITS OF THE GIFT OF QUIET CONTEMPLATION

_____

_____

_____

_____

_____

_____

_____

_____

> Enzyme-rich sprouted seeds are tiny power-houses of anti-inflammatory antioxidants and an outstanding source of many nutrients.

WEEK 1 / DAY 7   **DATE:** _____

BREAKFAST:

- 2 ounces lox
- 2 flax crackers
- 2 soft-boiled eggs
- ½ grapefruit
- 8 ounces green tea with lemon or spring water

Supplements:

- 1 packet of Weight Management supplements
- 1 1,000 mg fish oil capsule
- 1 astaxanthin capsule
- ½ teaspoon glutamine powder—mix in water and drink immediately

LUNCH:

- **Egyptian Chicken Salad***
- 1 apple
- 8 ounces spring water

Supplements:

- 1 packet of Weight Management supplements
- 1 1,000 mg fish oil capsule
- 1 astaxanthin capsule
- ½ teaspoon glutamine powder—mix in water and drink immediately

* All recipes can be found in *The Perricone Weight-Loss Diet*

Adding fiber to the diet helps regulate blood sugar levels, important in avoiding diabetes, metabolic disorders, and unwanted weight gain.

SNACK:

- ½ cup plain yogurt topped with 1 tablespoon POM Wonderful pomegranate juice or pure açaí pulp
- 2 tablespoons sesame seeds
- ⅓ cup blueberries
- 8 ounces spring water

DINNER:

- **Pan-Roasted Salmon with Wilted Chard and Tomato-Mint Raita***
- 1 cup of salad (dark green leafy lettuce, dressed with 1 tablespoon extra virgin olive oil; fresh lemon juice to taste)
- 1 pear
- 8 ounces white or green tea with lemon, or spring water

Supplements:

- 1 packet of Weight Management supplements
- 1 1,000 mg fish oil capsule
- 1 astaxanthin capsule
- ½ teaspoon glutamine powder—mix in water and drink immediately

BEDTIME:

- ½ cup cottage cheese with 1 diced apple and 4 slivered almonds
- 8 ounces spring water

* All recipes can be found in *The Perricone Weight-Loss Diet*

JOURNAL NOTES

THREE THINGS TO CELEBRATE FROM MY DAY:

1. _____

2. _____

3. _____

RECORD THE POSITIVE CHANGES
YOUR BODY EXPERIENCES EACH DAY

Weight: _____   Tone: _____

Energy: _____

Exercise: _____

RECORD THE POSITIVE MENTAL AND
EMOTIONAL EXPERIENCES EACH DAY

Changes in mood: _____

Stress handling: _____

Memory: _____

Problem-solving ability: _____

EMBRACING THE ANTI-INFLAMMATORY LIFESTYLE

Progress in overcoming bad habits:

_____

Progress in minimizing stress:

_____

Cups of coffee: _____   Alcohol: _____

Smoking: _____   Conflict/Tension: _____

Sleep (# of hours): _____   Sleep quality: _____

BENEFITS OF THE GIFT OF QUIET CONTEMPLATION

_____

_____

_____

_____

_____

_____

_____

_____

> Eat the skins of your fruits and vegetables if they
> are organic and unwaxed; the most fiber
> and greatest antioxidant/anti-inflammatory
> properties are in the skin.

WEEK 2 / DAY 8   DATE: _____

BREAKFAST:

- ½ cup cooked old-fashioned oatmeal, topped with 2 tablespoons yogurt, ¼ cup blueberries and 2 tablespoons sesame seeds
- 3 slices soy or turkey bacon
- 8 ounces green tea or spring water

Supplements:

- 1 packet of Weight Management supplements
- 1 1,000 mg fish oil capsule
- 1 astaxanthin capsule
- ½ teaspoon glutamine powder—mix in water and drink immediately

LUNCH:

- Halibut or salmon fillet, grilled, poached, or steamed (4–6 ounces raw weight boneless)
- **Miso Soup with Wilted Greens and Roasted Tomatoes***
- 1 pear
- 8 ounces green tea or spring water

Supplements:

- 1 packet of Weight Management supplements
- 1 1,000 mg fish oil capsule
- 1 astaxanthin capsule
- ½ teaspoon glutamine powder—mix in water and drink immediately

* All recipes can be found in *The Perricone Weight-Loss Diet*

> Fats with anti-inflammatory action are mono or polyunsaturated, and include extra virgin olive oil and foods rich in essential fatty acids (salmon, coconut, avocados, açaí, olives, nuts and seeds).

SNACK:

- ½ cup cottage cheese with 2 tablespoons salsa and 2 teaspoons sesame seeds
- 8 ounces spring water

DINNER:

- **Curried Stew*** with chicken, turkey, or tofu
- 1 cup of salad (dark green leafy lettuce, dressed with 1 tablespoon extra virgin olive oil; fresh lemon juice to taste)
- ½ cup mixed berries
- 8 ounces spring water

Supplements:

- 1 packet of Weight Management supplements
- 1 1,000 mg fish oil capsule
- 1 astaxanthin capsule
- ½ teaspoon glutamine powder—mix in water and drink immediately

BEDTIME:

- 1 hard-boiled egg
- Celery sticks and 2 tablespoons hummus
- 8 ounces spring water

* All recipes can be found in *The Perricone Weight-Loss Diet*

JOURNAL NOTES

THREE THINGS TO CELEBRATE FROM MY DAY:

1. _____

2. _____

3. _____

RECORD THE POSITIVE CHANGES
YOUR BODY EXPERIENCES EACH DAY

Weight: _____   Tone: _____

Energy: _____

Exercise: _____

RECORD THE POSITIVE MENTAL AND
EMOTIONAL EXPERIENCES EACH DAY

Changes in mood: _____

Stress handling: _____

Memory: _____

Problem-solving ability: _____

EMBRACING THE ANTI-INFLAMMATORY LIFESTYLE

Progress in overcoming bad habits:

_____

Progress in minimizing stress:

_____

Cups of coffee: _____   Alcohol: _____

Smoking: _____   Conflict/Tension: _____

Sleep (# of hours): _____   Sleep quality: _____

BENEFITS OF THE GIFT OF QUIET CONTEMPLATION

_____

_____

_____

_____

_____

_____

_____

_____

> A simple rule of thumb is to consider the
> following: if it contains flour, and/or sugar or
> other sweetener it will be pro-inflammatory.

WEEK 2 / DAY 9   DATE: _____

BREAKFAST:

♦ 2 whole eggs plus 1 egg white omelet with 3 tablespoons **Baba Ghanouj***

♦ 6 cherry tomatoes, halved and 1 teaspoon chopped cilantro

♦ ¾ cup plain yogurt with 2 tablespoons chopped almonds and ¼ teaspoon pure vanilla extract

♦ ½ grapefruit

♦ 8 ounces white or green tea or spring water

Supplements:

♦ 1 packet of Weight Management supplements

♦ 1 1,000 mg fish oil capsule

♦ 1 astaxanthin capsule

♦ ½ teaspoon glutamine powder—mix in water and drink immediately

LUNCH:

♦ **Tomato Avocado Soup with Fresh Crabmeat***

♦ 1 cup of salad (dark green leafy lettuce, dressed with 1 tablespoon extra virgin olive oil; fresh lemon juice to taste)

♦ ½ cup black raspberries

♦ 8 ounces iced green tea with lemon, or spring water

Supplements:

♦ 1 packet of Weight Management supplements

♦ 1 1,000 mg fish oil capsule

♦ 1 astaxanthin capsule

♦ ½ teaspoon glutamine powder—mix in water and drink immediately

*All recipes can be found in *The Perricone Weight-Loss Diet*

> An apple a day . . . a recent study showed that eating three small apples or pears per day appears to accelerate weight loss in women.

SNACK:

- Smoothie with ½ cup kefir, ¼ cup almond milk, and 6 (pitted) cherries
- 8 ounces spring water

DINNER:

- Grilled chicken (or salmon) (6–9 ounces raw weight boneless skinless) with **Pomegranate Walnut Sauce***
- Steamed kale
- 1 sliced pear
- 8 ounces **Moroccan Mint Tea*** or spring water

Supplements:

- 1 packet of Weight Management supplements
- 1 1,000 mg fish oil capsule
- 1 astaxanthin capsule
- ½ teaspoon glutamine powder—mix in water and drink immediately

BEDTIME:

- 2 ounces thinly sliced turkey breast
- 4 almonds
- 1 2-inch wedge honeydew
- 8 ounces spring water

* All recipes can be found in *The Perricone Weight-Loss Diet*

JOURNAL NOTES

THREE THINGS TO CELEBRATE FROM MY DAY:

1. _____

2. _____

3. _____

RECORD THE POSITIVE CHANGES
YOUR BODY EXPERIENCES EACH DAY

Weight: _____   Tone: _____

Energy: _____

Exercise: _____

RECORD THE POSITIVE MENTAL AND
EMOTIONAL EXPERIENCES EACH DAY

Changes in mood: _____

Stress handling: _____

Memory: _____

Problem-solving ability: _____

EMBRACING THE ANTI-INFLAMMATORY LIFESTYLE

Progress in overcoming bad habits:

_____

Progress in minimizing stress:

_____

Cups of coffee: _____   Alcohol: _____

Smoking: _____   Conflict/Tension: _____

Sleep (# of hours): _____   Sleep quality: _____

BENEFITS OF THE GIFT OF QUIET CONTEMPLATION

_____

_____

_____

_____

_____

_____

_____

_____

_____

> Try sugar-free salsa. Salsas contain hot peppers whose active ingredient, capsaicin, speeds up the body's metabolism and stimulates the production of saliva, which stimulates the digestive process.

WEEK 2 / DAY 10   **DATE:** _____

BREAKFAST:

♦ 3 egg omelet made with 2 egg whites, 1 whole egg, ¼ cup chopped roasted bell pepper, 2 tablespoons sautéed red onion and 1 teaspoon chopped basil

♦ ½ cup (measured dry) **Stop the Clock! Cereal*** cooked with water and ½ teaspoon ground cinnamon

♦ ½ cup fresh blueberries

♦ 8 ounces green tea or spring water

Supplements:

♦ 1 packet of Weight Management supplements

♦ 1 1,000 mg fish oil capsule

♦ 1 astaxanthin capsule

♦ ½ teaspoon glutamine powder—mix in water and drink immediately

LUNCH:

♦ **Asian Salad*** with 6 ounces grilled tofu or chicken breast

♦ ½ grapefruit

♦ 8 ounces iced green tea with lemon, or spring water

Supplements:

♦ 1 packet of Weight Management supplements

♦ 1 1,000 mg fish oil capsule

♦ 1 astaxanthin capsule

♦ ½ teaspoon glutamine powder—mix in water and drink immediately

* All recipes can be found in *The Perricone Weight-Loss Diet*

> Anti-inflammatory foods encourage the burning of fat for energy, eliminate food cravings, and do not stimulate the appetite.

SNACK:

♦ ½ cup plain yogurt with 1 tablespoon sesame seeds and 1 tablespoon pure açaí pulp or POM Wonderful pomegranate juice

♦ 8 ounces spring water

DINNER:

♦ **Three-Fish Etouffée with Baby Artichokes and Spicy Tomato Broth***

♦ 1 cup of salad (dark green leafy lettuce, dressed with 1 tablespoon extra virgin olive oil; fresh lemon juice to taste)

♦ 1 apple

♦ 8 ounces white tea with ginger slice, or spring water

Supplements:

♦ 1 packet of Weight Management supplements

♦ 1 1,000 mg fish oil capsule

♦ 1 astaxanthin capsule

♦ ½ teaspoon glutamine powder—mix in water and drink immediately

BEDTIME:

♦ Smoothie with ½ cup kefir, 2 tablespoons blackberries and 1 tablespoon POM Wonderful pomegranate juice or pure açaí pulp

♦ 8 ounces spring water

* All recipes can be found in *The Perricone Weight-Loss Diet*

JOURNAL NOTES

THREE THINGS TO CELEBRATE FROM MY DAY:

1. _____

2. _____

3. _____

RECORD THE POSITIVE CHANGES
YOUR BODY EXPERIENCES EACH DAY

Weight: _____   Tone: _____

Energy: _____

Exercise: _____

RECORD THE POSITIVE MENTAL AND
EMOTIONAL EXPERIENCES EACH DAY

Changes in mood: _____

Stress handling: _____

Memory: _____

Problem-solving ability: _____

EMBRACING THE ANTI-INFLAMMATORY LIFESTYLE

Progress in overcoming bad habits:

_____

Progress in minimizing stress:

_____

Cups of coffee: _____   Alcohol: _____

Smoking: _____   Conflict/Tension: _____

Sleep (# of hours): _____   Sleep quality: _____

BENEFITS OF THE GIFT OF QUIET CONTEMPLATION

_____

_____

_____

_____

_____

_____

_____

_____

_____

> Add some sesame seeds to your salad—studies show they promote fat burning.

WEEK 2 / DAY 11   DATE: _____

BREAKFAST:

- 2 eggs scrambled with 2 ounces sliced smoked salmon and 1 teaspoon chopped chives
- ¼ cup (measured dry) **Stop the Clock! Cereal*** with ¼ teaspoon ground ginger
- ½ cup sliced strawberries
- 8 ounces green tea or spring water

Supplements:

- 1 packet of Weight Management supplements
- 1 1,000 mg fish oil capsule
- 1 astaxanthin capsule
- ½ teaspoon glutamine powder—mix in water and drink immediately

LUNCH:

- Grilled sesame tofu or chicken (6 ounces)
- **Tomato-Ginger Bisque***
- 1 sliced kiwi
- 8 ounces spring water

Supplements:

- 1 packet of Weight Management supplements
- 1 1,000 mg fish oil capsule
- 1 astaxanthin capsule
- ½ teaspoon glutamine powder—mix in water and drink immediately

* All recipes can be found in *The Perricone Weight-Loss Diet*

> Exercise not only helps us to lose weight and gain muscle, it is also proven as a stress reducer and mood elevator.

SNACK:

♦ ½ cup cottage cheese with 1 teaspoon flaxseed and ⅓ cup diced apple

♦ 8 ounces spring water

DINNER:

♦ **Salmon Chermoula***

♦ 1 cup of salad (dark green leafy lettuce, dressed with 1 tablespoon extra virgin olive oil; fresh lemon juice to taste)

♦ 1 cup steamed broccoli

♦ 1 Asian pear

♦ 8 ounces spring water

Supplements:

♦ 1 packet of Weight Management supplements

♦ 1 1,000 mg fish oil capsule

♦ 1 astaxanthin capsule

♦ ½ teaspoon glutamine powder—mix in water and drink immediately

BEDTIME:

♦ 1 ounce sliced turkey

♦ ¼ avocado

♦ 8 ounces spring water

* All recipes can be found in *The Perricone Weight-Loss Diet*

JOURNAL NOTES

THREE THINGS TO CELEBRATE FROM MY DAY:

1. _____

2. _____

3. _____

RECORD THE POSITIVE CHANGES
YOUR BODY EXPERIENCES EACH DAY

Weight: _____   Tone: _____

Energy: _____

Exercise: _____

RECORD THE POSITIVE MENTAL AND
EMOTIONAL EXPERIENCES EACH DAY

Changes in mood: _____

Stress handling: _____

Memory: _____

Problem-solving ability: _____

EMBRACING THE ANTI-INFLAMMATORY LIFESTYLE

Progress in overcoming bad habits:

_____

Progress in minimizing stress:

_____

Cups of coffee: _____   Alcohol: _____

Smoking: _____   Conflict/Tension: _____

Sleep (# of hours): _____   Sleep quality: _____

BENEFITS OF THE GIFT OF QUIET CONTEMPLATION

_____

_____

_____

_____

_____

_____

_____

_____

> **Find ways to minimize stress because it promotes weight gain.**

WEEK 2 / DAY 12   DATE: _____

BREAKFAST:

- Grilled salmon fillet (4 ounces raw weight boneless)
- 6 cherry tomatoes
- ⅓ cup sliced strawberries
- 8 ounces green tea or spring water

Supplements:

- 1 packet of Weight Management supplements
- 1 1,000 mg fish oil capsule
- 1 astaxanthin capsule
- ½ teaspoon glutamine powder—mix in water and drink immediately

LUNCH:

- Grilled chicken breast (6 ounces raw weight boneless skinless) or tofu veggie burger
- 1 cup **Watercress and Almond Salad with Roasted Onion Dressing***
- ½ cup cherries
- 8 ounces spring water

Supplements:

- 1 packet of Weight Management supplements
- 1 1,000 mg fish oil capsule
- 1 astaxanthin capsule
- ½ teaspoon glutamine powder—mix in water and drink immediately

* All recipes can be found in *The Perricone Weight-Loss Diet*

> **Chronic, high stress levels cause us to overeat and to store fat in the abdominal region.**

SNACK:

- ♦ 1 ounce sliced chicken or turkey breast
- ♦ 4 almonds
- ♦ 1 apple
- ♦ 8 ounces spring water

DINNER:

- ♦ Salmon, trout, or mackerel (4–6 ounces raw weight boneless) with **Baba Ghanouj***
- ♦ Green beans sautéed with garlic and sesame oil
- ♦ 1 cup of salad (dark green leafy lettuce, dressed with 1 tablespoon extra virgin olive oil; fresh lemon juice to taste)
- ♦ Sliced pear
- ♦ 8 ounces green or white tea or spring water

Supplements:

- ♦ 1 packet of Weight Management supplements
- ♦ 1 1,000 mg fish oil capsule
- ♦ 1 astaxanthin capsule
- ♦ ½ teaspoon glutamine powder—mix in water and drink immediately

BEDTIME:

- ♦ ½ cup yogurt with 1 tablespoon POM Wonderful pomegranate juice or pure açaí pulp
- ♦ 4 almonds
- ♦ 1 peach
- ♦ 8 ounces spring water

* All recipes can be found in *The Perricone Weight-Loss Diet*

JOURNAL NOTES

THREE THINGS TO CELEBRATE FROM MY DAY:

1. _____

2. _____

3. _____

RECORD THE POSITIVE CHANGES
YOUR BODY EXPERIENCES EACH DAY

Weight: _____   Tone: _____

Energy: _____

Exercise: _____

RECORD THE POSITIVE MENTAL AND
EMOTIONAL EXPERIENCES EACH DAY

Changes in mood: _____

Stress handling: _____

Memory: _____

Problem-solving ability: _____

EMBRACING THE ANTI-INFLAMMATORY LIFESTYLE

Progress in overcoming bad habits:

_____

Progress in minimizing stress:

_____

Cups of coffee: _____   Alcohol: _____

Smoking: _____   Conflict/Tension: _____

Sleep (# of hours): _____   Sleep quality: _____

BENEFITS OF THE GIFT OF QUIET CONTEMPLATION

_____

_____

_____

_____

_____

_____

_____

_____

_____

Laughter is an excellent antidote to stress—it can lower levels of stress hormones, boost the immune system, and increase feelings of well being.

WEEK 2 / DAY 13

DATE: _____

BREAKFAST:

♦ 2 egg omelette with ½ ounce feta cheese, 3 cherry tomatoes, halved, and 1 teaspoon chopped green onion

♦ 2 links turkey sausage

♦ ½ cup blueberries

♦ 3 almonds

♦ 8 ounces spring water

Supplements:

♦ 1 packet of Weight Management supplements

♦ 1 1,000 mg fish oil capsule

♦ 1 astaxanthin capsule

♦ ½ teaspoon glutamine powder—mix in water and drink immediately

LUNCH:

♦ **Caribbean Fish Burger*** over baby greens

♦ ½ cup sliced tomatoes

♦ ¼ cup **Edamame Guacamole*** or ¼ sliced avocado

♦ ½ cup black raspberries

♦ 8 ounces iced green or white tea or spring water

Supplements:

♦ 1 packet of Weight Management supplements

♦ 1 1,000 mg fish oil capsule

♦ 1 astaxanthin capsule

♦ ½ teaspoon glutamine powder—mix in water and drink immediately

* All recipes can be found in *The Perricone Weight-Loss Diet*

> Studies show that green tea prevents the absorption of fat, helping to keep excess body fat under control.

SNACK:

♦ 1 ounce sliced turkey

♦ 2 flax crackers

♦ 2-inch slice honeydew

♦ 8 ounces spring water

DINNER:

♦ Salmon/fish **Mole with Pumpkin and Sunflower Seeds***

♦ Steamed artichoke

♦ 1 cup of salad (dark green leafy lettuce, dressed with 1 tablespoon extra virgin olive oil; fresh lemon juice to taste)

♦ 1 apple

♦ 8 ounces green tea or spring water

Supplements:

♦ 1 packet of Weight Management supplements

♦ 1 1,000 mg fish oil capsule

♦ 1 astaxanthin capsule

♦ ½ teaspoon glutamine powder—mix in water and drink immediately

BEDTIME:

♦ ½ cup cottage cheese topped with 1 tablespoon sesame seeds

♦ 1 pear

♦ 8 ounces spring water

* All recipes can be found in *The Perricone Weight-Loss Diet*

JOURNAL NOTES

THREE THINGS TO CELEBRATE FROM MY DAY:

1. _____

2. _____

3. _____

RECORD THE POSITIVE CHANGES
YOUR BODY EXPERIENCES EACH DAY

Weight: _____   Tone: _____

Energy: _____

Exercise: _____

RECORD THE POSITIVE MENTAL AND
EMOTIONAL EXPERIENCES EACH DAY

Changes in mood: _____

Stress handling: _____

Memory: _____

Problem-solving ability: _____

EMBRACING THE ANTI-INFLAMMATORY LIFESTYLE

Progress in overcoming bad habits:

_____

Progress in minimizing stress:

_____

Cups of coffee: _____   Alcohol: _____

Smoking: _____   Conflict/Tension: _____

Sleep (# of hours): _____   Sleep quality: _____

BENEFITS OF THE GIFT OF QUIET CONTEMPLATION

_____

_____

_____

_____

_____

_____

_____

_____

_____

> Choose brightly colored fruits and vegetables because they are high in antioxidants, nature's anti-inflammatories.

WEEK 2 / DAY 14   DATE: _____

BREAKFAST:

- 2 eggs, scrambled with chopped green onion and bell pepper
- 1 ounce lox
- ½ cup (measured dry) **Stop the Clock! Cereal*** with 1 teaspoon flax seed and 1 tablespoon sesame seeds
- ½ grapefruit
- 8 ounces green or white tea with fresh lemon or spring water

Supplements:

- 1 packet of Weight Management supplements
- 1 1,000 mg fish oil capsule
- 1 astaxanthin capsule
- ½ teaspoon glutamine powder—mix in water and drink immediately

LUNCH:

- **Sesame Seed-Encrusted Salmon***
- Arugula salad with extra virgin olive oil, fresh lemon juice, 3 sliced olives, and 4 cherry tomatoes
- 1 pear
- 8 ounces spring water

Supplements:

- 1 packet of Weight Management supplements
- 1 1,000 mg fish oil capsule
- 1 astaxanthin capsule
- ½ teaspoon glutamine powder—mix in water and drink immediately

* All recipes can be found in *The Perricone Weight-Loss Diet*

> For optimum benefits, exercise needs to be done on a regular basis.

SNACK:

- 1 ounce sliced smoked turkey
- 4 walnuts
- 1 apple
- 8 ounces spring water

DINNER:

- **Spicy Fish Stew***
- Wilted spinach or escarole with fresh lemon juice
- 1 cup of salad (dark green leafy lettuce, dressed with 1 tablespoon extra virgin olive oil; fresh lemon juice to taste)
- ½ cup berries
- 8 ounces spring water

Supplements:

- 1 packet of Weight Management supplements
- 1 1,000 mg fish oil capsule
- 1 astaxanthin capsule
- ½ teaspoon glutamine powder—mix in water and drink immediately

BEDTIME:

- Smoothie with ½ cup kefir, 6 cherries, and 1 tablespoon POM Wonderful pomegranate juice or pure açaí pulp

* All recipes can be found in *The Perricone Weight-Loss Diet*

JOURNAL NOTES

THREE THINGS TO CELEBRATE FROM MY DAY:

1. _____

2. _____

3. _____

RECORD THE POSITIVE CHANGES
YOUR BODY EXPERIENCES EACH DAY

Weight: _____   Tone: _____

Energy: _____

Exercise: _____

RECORD THE POSITIVE MENTAL AND
EMOTIONAL EXPERIENCES EACH DAY

Changes in mood: _____

Stress handling: _____

Memory: _____

Problem-solving ability: _____

EMBRACING THE ANTI-INFLAMMATORY LIFESTYLE

Progress in overcoming bad habits:

_____

Progress in minimizing stress:

_____

Cups of coffee: _____   Alcohol: _____

Smoking: _____   Conflict/Tension: _____

Sleep (# of hours): _____   Sleep quality: _____

BENEFITS OF THE GIFT OF QUIET CONTEMPLATION

_____

_____

_____

_____

_____

_____

_____

_____

_____

> **Always remember to eat the protein first at every meal.**

WEEK 3 / DAY 15   DATE: _____

BREAKFAST:

- 2 poached omega-3 eggs with **Indian Spinach***
- 2 slices turkey bacon
- ½ cup honeydew with 1 teaspoon chopped fresh mint
- 8 ounces green tea with slice of ginger or spring water

Supplements:

- 1 packet of Weight Management supplements
- 1 1,000 mg fish oil capsule
- 1 astaxanthin capsule
- ½ teaspoon glutamine powder—mix in water and drink immediately

LUNCH:

- 1½ cups **African Groundnut Stew***
- 1 cup of salad (dark green leafy lettuce, dressed with 1 tablespoon extra virgin olive oil; fresh lemon juice to taste)
- ⅓ cup berries
- 8 ounces spring water

Supplements:

- 1 packet of Weight Management supplements
- 1 1,000 mg fish oil capsule
- 1 astaxanthin capsule
- ½ teaspoon glutamine powder—mix in water and drink immediately

* All recipes can be found in *The Perricone Weight-Loss Diet*

> **Animal fats are pro-inflammatory saturated fats, so use them in moderation.**

SNACK:

- ¼ cup **Edamame Guacamole*** + 1 teaspoon flaxseed served with celery and jicama sticks
- 8 ounces spring water

DINNER:

- Poached or grilled salmon (6–8 ounces raw weight) with **Spring Roll Salad***
- Steamed asparagus
- 2-inch wedge of cantaloupe
- 8 ounces spring water

Supplements:

- 1 packet of Weight Management supplements
- 1 1,000 mg fish oil capsule
- 1 astaxanthin capsule
- ½ teaspoon glutamine powder—mix in water and drink immediately

BEDTIME:

- ¼ cup plain yogurt with ½ teaspoon vanilla
- 1 teaspoon ground flax
- ¼ cup raspberries
- **Moroccan Mint Tea*** or spring water

* All recipes can be found in *The Perricone Weight-Loss Diet*

JOURNAL NOTES

THREE THINGS TO CELEBRATE FROM MY DAY:

1. _____

2. _____

3. _____

RECORD THE POSITIVE CHANGES
YOUR BODY EXPERIENCES EACH DAY

Weight: _____   Tone: _____

Energy: _____

Exercise: _____

RECORD THE POSITIVE MENTAL AND
EMOTIONAL EXPERIENCES EACH DAY

Changes in mood: _____

Stress handling: _____

Memory: _____

Problem-solving ability: _____

EMBRACING THE ANTI-INFLAMMATORY LIFESTYLE

Progress in overcoming bad habits:

_____

Progress in minimizing stress:

_____

Cups of coffee: _____   Alcohol: _____

Smoking: _____   Conflict/Tension: _____

Sleep (# of hours): _____   Sleep quality: _____

BENEFITS OF THE GIFT OF QUIET CONTEMPLATION

_____

_____

_____

_____

_____

_____

_____

_____

_____

> Every meal or snack must include protein, low-glycemic carbs, and essential fatty acids.

WEEK 3 / DAY 16   DATE: _____

BREAKFAST:

- 2 soft-boiled eggs
- ½ cup (measured dry) **Stop the Clock! Cereal*** with 1 tablespoon POM Wonderful pomegranate juice or pure açaí pulp
- ½ cup plain yogurt with ½ cup diced cantaloupe and 1 teaspoon chopped mint
- 8 ounces green tea or spring water

Supplements:

- 1 packet of Weight Management supplements
- 1 1,000 mg fish oil capsule
- 1 astaxanthin capsule
- ½ teaspoon glutamine powder—mix in water and drink immediately

LUNCH:

- **Icy Gazpacho with Fresh Lime***
- Grilled chicken breast (6 ounces raw weight boneless skinless)
- 1 cup of salad (dark green leafy lettuce, dressed with 1 tablespoon extra virgin olive oil; fresh lemon juice to taste)
- ½ grapefruit
- 8 ounces iced green tea or spring water

Supplements:

- 1 packet of Weight Management supplements
- 1 1,000 mg fish oil capsule
- 1 astaxanthin capsule
- ½ teaspoon glutamine powder—mix in water and drink immediately

* All recipes can be found in *The Perricone Weight-Loss Diet*

> Omega-3 fatty acids found in fish and fish oil
> help us burn off calories before they get a
> chance to be stored as fat.

SNACK:

♦ ⅓ cup cottage cheese with 1 tablespoon ground flax and ¼ cup blueberries

♦ 8 ounces spring water

DINNER:

♦ Poached or baked halibut (or salmon) (6–8 ounces raw weight boneless) with **Curried Cabbage***

♦ 1 cup of cherry tomato salad with 1 teaspoon each chopped ginger, cilantro, extra virgin olive oil; low-sodium soy sauce and fresh lemon juice to taste

♦ 1 pear

♦ 8 ounces spring water with fresh lime

Supplements:

♦ 1 packet of Weight Management supplements

♦ 1 1,000 mg fish oil capsule

♦ 1 astaxanthin capsule

♦ ½ teaspoon glutamine powder—mix in water and drink immediately

BEDTIME:

♦ ½ cup kefir

♦ 3 almonds

♦ 6 cherries

♦ 8 ounces spring water

* All recipes can be found in *The Perricone Weight-Loss Diet*

JOURNAL NOTES

THREE THINGS TO CELEBRATE FROM MY DAY:

1. _____

2. _____

3. _____

RECORD THE POSITIVE CHANGES
YOUR BODY EXPERIENCES EACH DAY

Weight: _____   Tone: _____

Energy: _____

Exercise: _____

RECORD THE POSITIVE MENTAL AND
EMOTIONAL EXPERIENCES EACH DAY

Changes in mood: _____

Stress handling: _____

Memory: _____

Problem-solving ability: _____

EMBRACING THE ANTI-INFLAMMATORY LIFESTYLE

Progress in overcoming bad habits:

_____

Progress in minimizing stress:

_____

Cups of coffee: _____   Alcohol: _____

Smoking: _____   Conflict/Tension: _____

Sleep (# of hours): _____   Sleep quality: _____

BENEFITS OF THE GIFT OF QUIET CONTEMPLATION

_____

_____

_____

_____

_____

_____

_____

_____

_____

> **Always eat your protein first.**
> **This will help suppress your appetite.**

WEEK 3 / DAY 17   DATE: _____

BREAKFAST:

♦   2 whole eggs plus two egg whites scrambled with 1 slice turkey bacon and **Nutty Tomato Pesto***

♦   ½ grapefruit

♦   8 ounces green tea or spring water

Supplements:

♦   1 packet of Weight Management supplements

♦   1 1,000 mg fish oil capsule

♦   1 astaxanthin capsule

♦   ½ teaspoon glutamine powder—mix in water and drink immediately

LUNCH:

♦   Salmon fillet, baked or grilled (4–6 ounces raw weight boneless) with 1 cup **Caponata*** salad served on mixed baby greens

♦   ½ cup raspberries

♦   8 ounces iced white or green tea or spring water

Supplements:

♦   1 packet of Weight Management supplements

♦   1 1,000 mg fish oil capsule

♦   1 astaxanthin capsule

♦   ½ teaspoon glutamine powder—mix in water and drink immediately

* All recipes can be found in *The Perricone Weight-Loss Diet*

A good night's sleep can help you wake
refreshed, looking radiant and youthful.
And, after a good night's sleep, doesn't the
world look better, too?

SNACK:

♦ Smoothie with ½ cup kefir, 1 teaspoon ground flax, and ½ cup sliced strawberries

♦ 8 ounces spring water

DINNER:

♦ Grilled shrimp (6 ounces raw weight)

♦ **Scalloped Tomatoes with Caramelized Onions***

♦ 1 cup of salad (dark green leafy lettuce, dressed with 1 tablespoon extra virgin olive oil; fresh lemon juice to taste)

♦ 1 apple

♦ 8 ounces spring water

Supplements:

♦ 1 packet of Weight Management supplements

♦ 1 1,000 mg fish oil capsule

♦ 1 astaxanthin capsule

♦ ½ teaspoon glutamine powder—mix in water and drink immediately

BEDTIME:

♦ 1 ounce sliced smoked salmon with 2 flax crackers

♦ 1 kiwi

♦ 8 ounces spring water

* All recipes can be found in *The Perricone Weight-Loss Diet*

JOURNAL NOTES

THREE THINGS TO CELEBRATE FROM MY DAY:

1. _____

2. _____

3. _____

RECORD THE POSITIVE CHANGES
YOUR BODY EXPERIENCES EACH DAY

Weight: _____   Tone: _____

Energy: _____

Exercise: _____

RECORD THE POSITIVE MENTAL AND
EMOTIONAL EXPERIENCES EACH DAY

Changes in mood: _____

Stress handling: _____

Memory: _____

Problem-solving ability: _____

EMBRACING THE ANTI-INFLAMMATORY LIFESTYLE

Progress in overcoming bad habits:

_____

Progress in minimizing stress:

_____

Cups of coffee: _____   Alcohol: _____

Smoking: _____   Conflict/Tension: _____

Sleep (# of hours): _____   Sleep quality: _____

BENEFITS OF THE GIFT OF QUIET CONTEMPLATION

_____

_____

_____

_____

_____

_____

_____

_____

> **Save the fresh fruit for the end of the meal. This will prevent the natural sugars found in the fruit from causing a spike in blood sugar.**

WEEK 3 / DAY 18   DATE: _____

BREAKFAST:
- 1 boiled egg
- ½ cup **Stop the Clock! Cereal***
- ½ cup **Blueberry Compote*** with 1 cup plain yogurt
- 8 ounces green or white tea or spring water

Supplements:
- 1 packet of Weight Management supplements
- 1 1,000 mg fish oil capsule
- 1 astaxanthin capsule
- ½ teaspoon glutamine powder—mix in water and drink immediately

LUNCH:
- Grilled turkey burger (4–6 ounces raw weight) served on baby spinach
- Tossed green salad with ¼ avocado slice
- 1 apple
- 8 ounces iced green tea with lemon or spring water

Supplements:
- 1 packet of Weight Management supplements
- 1 1,000 mg fish oil capsule
- 1 astaxanthin capsule
- ½ teaspoon glutamine powder—mix in water and drink immediately

* All recipes can be found in *The Perricone Weight-Loss Diet*

> **Essential fatty acids found in fish and fish oil lower insulin levels. High levels of insulin cause weight gain and block weight loss.**

SNACK:

♦ Cantaloupe wedge wrapped with 1 ounce slice of turkey breast, drizzled with 1 teaspoon flax oil

♦ 8 ounces spring water

DINNER:

♦ Grilled salmon (6–8 ounces raw weight) with **Creamy Onion Sauce with Roasted Garlic and Thyme***

♦ Steamed artichoke

♦ 1 cup of salad (dark green leafy lettuce, dressed with 1 tablespoon extra virgin olive oil; fresh lemon juice to taste)

♦ 8 ounces spring water

Supplements:

♦ 1 packet of Weight Management supplements

♦ 1 1,000 mg fish oil capsule

♦ 1 astaxanthin capsule

♦ ½ teaspoon glutamine powder—mix in water and drink immediately

BEDTIME:

♦ ¼ cup yogurt mixed with 1 tablespoon POM Wonderful pomegranate juice or pure açaí pulp

♦ 2 tablespoons sliced almonds

♦ ½ kiwi, diced

♦ 8 ounces spring water

* All recipes can be found in *The Perricone Weight-Loss Diet*

JOURNAL NOTES

THREE THINGS TO CELEBRATE FROM MY DAY:

1. _____

2. _____

3. _____

RECORD THE POSITIVE CHANGES
YOUR BODY EXPERIENCES EACH DAY

Weight: _____   Tone: _____

Energy: _____

Exercise: _____

RECORD THE POSITIVE MENTAL AND
EMOTIONAL EXPERIENCES EACH DAY

Changes in mood: _____

Stress handling: _____

Memory: _____

Problem-solving ability: _____

EMBRACING THE ANTI-INFLAMMATORY LIFESTYLE

Progress in overcoming bad habits:

_____

Progress in minimizing stress:

_____

Cups of coffee: _____   Alcohol: _____

Smoking: _____   Conflict/Tension: _____

Sleep (# of hours): _____   Sleep quality: _____

BENEFITS OF THE GIFT OF QUIET CONTEMPLATION

_____

_____

_____

_____

_____

_____

_____

_____

_____

> Looking for a fat-burner, muscle-builder, wrinkle-eraser, skin-saver, depression-lifter, and brain-booster? Try wild Alaskan salmon!

WEEK 3 / DAY 19   DATE: _____

BREAKFAST:

- 2 egg omelet with 2 ounces smoked salmon, fresh dill, and cherry tomatoes
- ⅓ cup kefir with 2 tablespoons blackberries
- 8 ounces green or white tea or spring water

Supplements:

- 1 packet of Weight Management supplements
- 1 1,000 mg fish oil capsule
- 1 astaxanthin capsule
- ½ teaspoon glutamine powder—mix in water and drink immediately

LUNCH:

- 6 ounces **Egyptian Chicken Salad***
- 1 cup **Broccoli Dill Soup with Lemon and Tahini***
- 1 apple
- 8 ounces spring water

Supplements:

- 1 packet of Weight Management supplements
- 1 1,000 mg fish oil capsule
- 1 astaxanthin capsule
- ½ teaspoon glutamine powder—mix in water and drink immediately

* All recipes can be found in *The Perricone Weight-Loss Diet*

> Our goal is to avoid spikes in blood sugar
> because they trigger insulin release.
> Remember this fact: insulin release = stored fat!

SNACK:

- ◆ ½ cup yogurt with 1 tablespoon chopped hazelnuts and ¼ cup diced kiwi
- ◆ 8 ounces spring water

DINNER:

- ◆ Grilled sablefish (or salmon) (6–8 ounces raw weight skinless)
- ◆ **Cucumber-Tomato Salad***
- ◆ **Brussels Sprouts with Slivered Almonds***
- ◆ 8 ounces spring water

Supplements:

- ◆ 1 packet of Weight Management supplements
- ◆ 1 1,000 mg fish oil capsule
- ◆ 1 astaxanthin capsule
- ◆ ½ teaspoon glutamine powder—mix in water and drink immediately

BEDTIME:

- ◆ ½ cup cottage cheese with 1 teaspoon ground flaxseed and ⅓ cup sliced strawberries
- ◆ 8 ounces spring water

* All recipes can be found in *The Perricone Weight-Loss Diet*

JOURNAL NOTES

THREE THINGS TO CELEBRATE FROM MY DAY:

1. _____

2. _____

3. _____

RECORD THE POSITIVE CHANGES
YOUR BODY EXPERIENCES EACH DAY

Weight: _____   Tone: _____

Energy: _____

Exercise: _____

RECORD THE POSITIVE MENTAL AND
EMOTIONAL EXPERIENCES EACH DAY

Changes in mood: _____

Stress handling: _____

Memory: _____

Problem-solving ability: _____

EMBRACING THE ANTI-INFLAMMATORY LIFESTYLE

Progress in overcoming bad habits:

_____

Progress in minimizing stress:

_____

Cups of coffee: _____   Alcohol: _____

Smoking: _____   Conflict/Tension: _____

Sleep (# of hours): _____   Sleep quality: _____

BENEFITS OF THE GIFT OF QUIET CONTEMPLATION

_____

_____

_____

_____

_____

_____

_____

_____

> **If you don't drink water,**
> **your body cannot metabolize fat.**

WEEK 3 / DAY 20   DATE: _____

BREAKFAST:

- ◆ 2 hard-boiled omega-3 eggs
- ◆ ½ cup (measured dry) **Stop the Clock! Cereal***
- ◆ ⅓ cup blueberries or blackberries plus ¼ cup plain yogurt
- ◆ 8 ounces green tea with lemon or spring water

Supplements:

- ◆ 1 packet of Weight Management supplements
- ◆ 1 1,000 mg fish oil capsule
- ◆ 1 astaxanthin capsule
- ◆ ½ teaspoon glutamine powder—mix in water and drink immediately

LUNCH:

- ◆ Poached or baked salmon (4–6 ounces raw weight boneless)
- ◆ 1 cup **Persian Vegetable Soup***
- ◆ 1 2-inch wedge honeydew
- ◆ 8 ounces spring water

Supplements:

- ◆ 1 packet of Weight Management supplements
- ◆ 1 1,000 mg fish oil capsule
- ◆ 1 astaxanthin capsule
- ◆ ½ teaspoon glutamine powder—mix in water and drink immediately

* All recipes can be found in *The Perricone Weight-Loss Diet*

> Eat raw foods for enzymes. Enzymes are critical to good health as they assist in the digestion and absorption of nutrients from food.

SNACK:

- Smoothie with ½ cup kefir, 1 teaspoon flax oil, pinch of cinnamon, and 2 tablespoons raspberries
- 8 ounces spring water

DINNER:

- **Grilled Miso Salmon (or Chicken)*** (6–8 ounces raw weight)
- Sautéed spinach (or escarole) and mushrooms
- 1 cup of salad (dark green leafy lettuce, dressed with 1 tablespoon extra virgin olive oil; fresh lemon juice to taste)
- 1 apple
- 8 ounces green tea or spring water

Supplements:

- 1 packet of Weight Management supplements
- 1 1,000 mg fish oil capsule
- 1 astaxanthin capsule
- ½ teaspoon glutamine powder—mix in water and drink immediately

BEDTIME:

- 1 ounce slice smoked chicken
- 4 walnuts
- 1 2-inch wedge honeydew
- 8 ounces spring water

* All recipes can be found in *The Perricone Weight-Loss Diet*

JOURNAL NOTES

THREE THINGS TO CELEBRATE FROM MY DAY:

1. _____

2. _____

3. _____

RECORD THE POSITIVE CHANGES
YOUR BODY EXPERIENCES EACH DAY

Weight: _____   Tone: _____

Energy: _____

Exercise: _____

RECORD THE POSITIVE MENTAL AND
EMOTIONAL EXPERIENCES EACH DAY

Changes in mood: _____

Stress handling: _____

Memory: _____

Problem-solving ability: _____

EMBRACING THE ANTI-INFLAMMATORY LIFESTYLE

Progress in overcoming bad habits:

_____

Progress in minimizing stress:

_____

Cups of coffee: _____   Alcohol: _____

Smoking: _____   Conflict/Tension: _____

Sleep (# of hours): _____   Sleep quality: _____

BENEFITS OF THE GIFT OF QUIET CONTEMPLATION

_____

_____

_____

_____

_____

_____

_____

_____

_____

> Enzyme-rich sprouted seeds are tiny power-houses of anti-inflammatory antioxidants and an outstanding source of many nutrients.

WEEK 3 / DAY 21   DATE: _____

BREAKFAST:

- 2 ounces lox
- 2 flax crackers
- 2 soft-boiled eggs
- ½ grapefruit
- 8 ounces green tea with lemon or spring water

Supplements:

- 1 packet of Weight Management supplements
- 1 1,000 mg fish oil capsule
- 1 astaxanthin capsule
- ½ teaspoon glutamine powder—mix in water and drink immediately

LUNCH:

- **Egyptian Chicken Salad***
- 1 apple
- 8 ounces spring water

Supplements:

- 1 packet of Weight Management supplements
- 1 1,000 mg fish oil capsule
- 1 astaxanthin capsule
- ½ teaspoon glutamine powder—mix in water and drink immediately

* All recipes can be found in *The Perricone Weight-Loss Diet*

> **Adding fiber to the diet helps regulate blood sugar levels, important in avoiding diabetes, metabolic disorders, and unwanted weight gain.**

SNACK:

♦ ½ cup plain yogurt topped with 1 tablespoon POM Wonderful pomegranate juice or pure açaí pulp

♦ 2 tablespoons sesame seeds

♦ ⅓ cup blueberries

♦ 8 ounces spring water

DINNER:

♦ **Pan-Roasted Salmon with Wilted Chard and Tomato-Mint Raita***

♦ 1 cup of salad (dark green leafy lettuce, dressed with 1 tablespoon extra virgin olive oil; fresh lemon juice to taste)

♦ 1 pear

♦ 8 ounces white or green tea with lemon, or spring water

Supplements:

♦ 1 packet of Weight Management supplements

♦ 1 1,000 mg fish oil capsule

♦ 1 astaxanthin capsule

♦ ½ teaspoon glutamine powder—mix in water and drink immediately

BEDTIME:

♦ ½ cup cottage cheese with 1 diced apple and 4 slivered almonds

♦ 8 ounces spring water

* All recipes can be found in *The Perricone Weight-Loss Diet*

JOURNAL NOTES

THREE THINGS TO CELEBRATE FROM MY DAY:

1. _____

2. _____

3. _____

RECORD THE POSITIVE CHANGES
YOUR BODY EXPERIENCES EACH DAY

Weight: _____   Tone: _____

Energy: _____

Exercise: _____

RECORD THE POSITIVE MENTAL AND
EMOTIONAL EXPERIENCES EACH DAY

Changes in mood: _____

Stress handling: _____

Memory: _____

Problem-solving ability: _____

EMBRACING THE ANTI-INFLAMMATORY LIFESTYLE

Progress in overcoming bad habits:

_____

Progress in minimizing stress:

_____

Cups of coffee: _____   Alcohol: _____

Smoking: _____   Conflict/Tension: _____

Sleep (# of hours): _____   Sleep quality: _____

BENEFITS OF THE GIFT OF QUIET CONTEMPLATION

_____

_____

_____

_____

_____

_____

_____

_____

_____

> **Eat the skins of your fruits and vegetables if they are organic and unwaxed; the most fiber and greatest antioxidant/anti-inflammatory properties are in the skin.**

WEEK 4 / DAY 22   DATE: _____

BREAKFAST:

♦ ½ cup cooked old-fashioned oatmeal, topped with 2 tablespoons yogurt, ¼ cup blueberries and 2 tablespoons sesame seeds

♦ 3 slices soy or turkey bacon

♦ 8 ounces green tea or spring water

Supplements:

♦ 1 packet of Weight Management supplements

♦ 1 1,000 mg fish oil capsule

♦ 1 astaxanthin capsule

♦ ½ teaspoon glutamine powder—mix in water and drink immediately

LUNCH:

♦ Halibut or salmon fillet, grilled, poached, or steamed (4–6 ounces raw weight boneless)

♦ **Miso Soup with Wilted Greens and Roasted Tomatoes***

♦ 1 pear

♦ 8 ounces green tea or spring water

Supplements:

♦ 1 packet of Weight Management supplements

♦ 1 1,000 mg fish oil capsule

♦ 1 astaxanthin capsule

♦ ½ teaspoon glutamine powder—mix in water and drink immediately

* All recipes can be found in *The Perricone Weight-Loss Diet*

> Fats with anti-inflammatory action are mono or polyunsaturated, and include extra virgin olive oil and foods rich in essential fatty acids (salmon, coconut, avocados, açaí, olives, nuts and seeds).

SNACK:

- ½ cup cottage cheese with 2 tablespoons salsa and 2 teaspoons sesame seeds
- 8 ounces spring water

DINNER:

- **Curried Stew*** with chicken, turkey, or tofu
- 1 cup of salad (dark green leafy lettuce, dressed with 1 tablespoon extra virgin olive oil; fresh lemon juice to taste)
- ½ cup mixed berries
- 8 ounces spring water

Supplements:

- 1 packet of Weight Management supplements
- 1 1,000 mg fish oil capsule
- 1 astaxanthin capsule
- ½ teaspoon glutamine powder—mix in water and drink immediately

BEDTIME:

- 1 hard-boiled egg
- Celery sticks and 2 tablespoons hummus
- 8 ounces spring water

* All recipes can be found in *The Perricone Weight-Loss Diet*

JOURNAL NOTES

THREE THINGS TO CELEBRATE FROM MY DAY:

1. _____

2. _____

3. _____

RECORD THE POSITIVE CHANGES
YOUR BODY EXPERIENCES EACH DAY

Weight: _____   Tone: _____

Energy: _____

Exercise: _____

RECORD THE POSITIVE MENTAL AND
EMOTIONAL EXPERIENCES EACH DAY

Changes in mood: _____

Stress handling: _____

Memory: _____

Problem-solving ability: _____

EMBRACING THE ANTI-INFLAMMATORY LIFESTYLE

Progress in overcoming bad habits:

_____

Progress in minimizing stress:

_____

Cups of coffee: _____   Alcohol: _____

Smoking: _____   Conflict/Tension: _____

Sleep (# of hours): _____   Sleep quality: _____

BENEFITS OF THE GIFT OF QUIET CONTEMPLATION

_____

_____

_____

_____

_____

_____

_____

_____

_____

> A simple rule of thumb is to consider the following: if it contains flour, and/or sugar or other sweetener it will be pro-inflammatory.

WEEK 4 / DAY 23   DATE: _____

BREAKFAST:

♦ 2 whole eggs plus 1 egg white omelet with 3 tablespoons **Baba Ghanouj***

♦ 6 cherry tomatoes, halved and 1 teaspoon chopped cilantro

♦ ¾ cup plain yogurt with 2 tablespoons chopped almonds and ¼ teaspoon pure vanilla extract

♦ ½ grapefruit

♦ 8 ounces white or green tea or spring water

Supplements:

♦ 1 packet of Weight Management supplements

♦ 1 1,000 mg fish oil capsule

♦ 1 astaxanthin capsule

♦ ½ teaspoon glutamine powder—mix in water and drink immediately

LUNCH:

♦ **Tomato Avocado Soup with Fresh Crabmeat***

♦ 1 cup of salad (dark green leafy lettuce, dressed with 1 tablespoon extra virgin olive oil; fresh lemon juice to taste)

♦ ½ cup black raspberries

♦ 8 ounces iced green tea with lemon, or spring water

Supplements:

♦ 1 packet of Weight Management supplements

♦ 1 1,000 mg fish oil capsule

♦ 1 astaxanthin capsule

♦ ½ teaspoon glutamine powder—mix in water and drink immediately

* All recipes can be found in *The Perricone Weight-Loss Diet*

An apple a day . . . a recent study showed that eating three small apples or pears per day appears to accelerate weight loss in women.

SNACK:

♦ Smoothie with ½ cup kefir, ¼ cup almond milk, and 6 (pitted) cherries

♦ 8 ounces spring water

DINNER:

♦ Grilled chicken (or salmon) (6–9 ounces raw weight boneless skinless) with **Pomegranate Walnut Sauce***

♦ Steamed kale

♦ 1 sliced pear

♦ 8 ounces **Moroccan Mint Tea*** or spring water

Supplements:

♦ 1 packet of Weight Management supplements

♦ 1 1,000 mg fish oil capsule

♦ 1 astaxanthin capsule

♦ ½ teaspoon glutamine powder—mix in water and drink immediately

BEDTIME:

♦ 2 ounces thinly sliced turkey breast

♦ 4 almonds

♦ 1 2-inch wedge honeydew

♦ 8 ounces spring water

* All recipes can be found in *The Perricone Weight-Loss Diet*

JOURNAL NOTES

THREE THINGS TO CELEBRATE FROM MY DAY:

1. _____

2. _____

3. _____

RECORD THE POSITIVE CHANGES
YOUR BODY EXPERIENCES EACH DAY

Weight: _____   Tone: _____

Energy: _____

Exercise: _____

RECORD THE POSITIVE MENTAL AND
EMOTIONAL EXPERIENCES EACH DAY

Changes in mood: _____

Stress handling: _____

Memory: _____

Problem-solving ability: _____

EMBRACING THE ANTI-INFLAMMATORY LIFESTYLE

Progress in overcoming bad habits:

_____

Progress in minimizing stress:

_____

Cups of coffee: _____   Alcohol: _____

Smoking: _____   Conflict/Tension: _____

Sleep (# of hours): _____   Sleep quality: _____

BENEFITS OF THE GIFT OF QUIET CONTEMPLATION

_____

_____

_____

_____

_____

_____

_____

_____

_____

> Try sugar-free salsa. Salsas contain hot peppers whose active ingredient, capsaicin, speeds up the body's metabolism and stimulates the production of saliva, which stimulates the digestive process.

WEEK 4 / DAY 24　　　　　**DATE:** _____

BREAKFAST:

♦ 3 egg omelet made with 2 egg whites, 1 whole egg, ¼ cup chopped roasted bell pepper, 2 tablespoons sautéed red onion and 1 teaspoon chopped basil

♦ ½ cup (measured dry) **Stop the Clock! Cereal*** cooked with water and ½ teaspoon ground cinnamon

♦ ½ cup fresh blueberries

♦ 8 ounces green tea or spring water

Supplements:

♦ 1 packet of Weight Management supplements

♦ 1 1,000 mg fish oil capsule

♦ 1 astaxanthin capsule

♦ ½ teaspoon glutamine powder—mix in water and drink immediately

LUNCH:

♦ **Asian Salad*** with 6 ounces grilled tofu or chicken breast

♦ ½ grapefruit

♦ 8 ounces iced green tea with lemon, or spring water

Supplements:

♦ 1 packet of Weight Management supplements

♦ 1 1,000 mg fish oil capsule

♦ 1 astaxanthin capsule

♦ ½ teaspoon glutamine powder—mix in water and drink immediately

* All recipes can be found in *The Perricone Weight-Loss Diet*

> Anti-inflammatory foods encourage the burning of fat for energy, eliminate food cravings, and do not stimulate the appetite.

SNACK:

♦ ½ cup plain yogurt with 1 tablespoon sesame seeds and 1 tablespoon pure açaí pulp or POM Wonderful pomegranate juice

♦ 8 ounces spring water

DINNER:

♦ **Three-Fish Etouffée with Baby Artichokes and Spicy Tomato Broth***

♦ 1 cup of salad (dark green leafy lettuce, dressed with 1 tablespoon extra virgin olive oil; fresh lemon juice to taste)

♦ 1 apple

♦ 8 ounces white tea with ginger slice, or spring water

Supplements:

♦ 1 packet of Weight Management supplements

♦ 1 1,000 mg fish oil capsule

♦ 1 astaxanthin capsule

♦ ½ teaspoon glutamine powder—mix in water and drink immediately

BEDTIME:

♦ Smoothie with ½ cup kefir, 2 tablespoons blackberries and 1 tablespoon POM Wonderful pomegranate juice or pure açaí pulp

♦ 8 ounces spring water

* All recipes can be found in *The Perricone Weight-Loss Diet*

JOURNAL NOTES

THREE THINGS TO CELEBRATE FROM MY DAY:

1. _____

2. _____

3. _____

RECORD THE POSITIVE CHANGES
YOUR BODY EXPERIENCES EACH DAY

Weight: _____   Tone: _____

Energy: _____

Exercise: _____

RECORD THE POSITIVE MENTAL AND
EMOTIONAL EXPERIENCES EACH DAY

Changes in mood: _____

Stress handling: _____

Memory: _____

Problem-solving ability: _____

EMBRACING THE ANTI-INFLAMMATORY LIFESTYLE

Progress in overcoming bad habits:

_____

Progress in minimizing stress:

_____

Cups of coffee: _____   Alcohol: _____

Smoking: _____   Conflict/Tension: _____

Sleep (# of hours): _____   Sleep quality: _____

BENEFITS OF THE GIFT OF QUIET CONTEMPLATION

_____

_____

_____

_____

_____

_____

_____

_____

_____

> **Add some sesame seeds to your salad—studies show they promote fat burning.**

WEEK 4 / DAY 25   DATE: _____

BREAKFAST:

♦ 2 eggs scrambled with 2 ounces sliced smoked salmon and 1 teaspoon chopped chives

♦ ¼ cup (measured dry) **Stop the Clock! Cereal*** with ¼ teaspoon ground ginger

♦ ½ cup sliced strawberries

♦ 8 ounces green tea or spring water

Supplements:

♦ 1 packet of Weight Management supplements

♦ 1 1,000 mg fish oil capsule

♦ 1 astaxanthin capsule

♦ ½ teaspoon glutamine powder—mix in water and drink immediately

LUNCH:

♦ Grilled sesame tofu or chicken (6 ounces)

♦ **Tomato-Ginger Bisque***

♦ 1 sliced kiwi

♦ 8 ounces spring water

Supplements:

♦ 1 packet of Weight Management supplements

♦ 1 1,000 mg fish oil capsule

♦ 1 astaxanthin capsule

♦ ½ teaspoon glutamine powder—mix in water and drink immediately

* All recipes can be found in *The Perricone Weight-Loss Diet*

> Exercise not only helps us to lose weight and gain muscle, it is also proven as a stress reducer and mood elevator.

SNACK:

♦ ½ cup cottage cheese with 1 teaspoon flaxseed and ⅓ cup diced apple

♦ 8 ounces spring water

DINNER:

♦ **Salmon Chermoula***

♦ 1 cup of salad (dark green leafy lettuce, dressed with 1 tablespoon extra virgin olive oil; fresh lemon juice to taste)

♦ 1 cup steamed broccoli

♦ 1 Asian pear

♦ 8 ounces spring water

Supplements:

♦ 1 packet of Weight Management supplements

♦ 1 1,000 mg fish oil capsule

♦ 1 astaxanthin capsule

♦ ½ teaspoon glutamine powder—mix in water and drink immediately

BEDTIME:

♦ 1 ounce sliced turkey

♦ ¼ avocado

♦ 8 ounces spring water

* All recipes can be found in *The Perricone Weight-Loss Diet*

JOURNAL NOTES

THREE THINGS TO CELEBRATE FROM MY DAY:

1. _____

2. _____

3. _____

RECORD THE POSITIVE CHANGES
YOUR BODY EXPERIENCES EACH DAY

Weight: _____   Tone: _____

Energy: _____

Exercise: _____

RECORD THE POSITIVE MENTAL AND
EMOTIONAL EXPERIENCES EACH DAY

Changes in mood: _____

Stress handling: _____

Memory: _____

Problem-solving ability: _____

EMBRACING THE ANTI-INFLAMMATORY LIFESTYLE

Progress in overcoming bad habits:

_____

Progress in minimizing stress:

_____

Cups of coffee: _____   Alcohol: _____

Smoking: _____   Conflict/Tension: _____

Sleep (# of hours): _____   Sleep quality: _____

BENEFITS OF THE GIFT OF QUIET CONTEMPLATION

_____

_____

_____

_____

_____

_____

_____

_____

_____

> Find ways to minimize stress because it promotes weight gain.

WEEK 4 / DAY 26   **DATE:** _____

BREAKFAST:

♦ Grilled salmon fillet (4 ounces raw weight boneless)
♦ 6 cherry tomatoes
♦ ⅓ cup sliced strawberries
♦ 8 ounces green tea or spring water

Supplements:

♦ 1 packet of Weight Management supplements
♦ 1 1,000 mg fish oil capsule
♦ 1 astaxanthin capsule
♦ ½ teaspoon glutamine powder—mix in water and drink immediately

LUNCH:

♦ Grilled chicken breast (6 ounces raw weight boneless skinless) or tofu veggie burger
♦ 1 cup **Watercress and Almond Salad with Roasted Onion Dressing***
♦ ½ cup cherries
♦ 8 ounces spring water

Supplements:

♦ 1 packet of Weight Management supplements
♦ 1 1,000 mg fish oil capsule
♦ 1 astaxanthin capsule
♦ ½ teaspoon glutamine powder—mix in water and drink immediately

* All recipes can be found in *The Perricone Weight-Loss Diet*

> Chronic, high stress levels cause us to overeat and to store fat in the abdominal region.

SNACK:

♦ 1 ounce sliced chicken or turkey breast

♦ 4 almonds

♦ 1 apple

♦ 8 ounces spring water

DINNER:

♦ Salmon, trout, or mackerel (4–6 ounces raw weight boneless) with **Baba Ghanouj***

♦ Green beans sautéed with garlic and sesame oil

♦ 1 cup of salad (dark green leafy lettuce, dressed with 1 tablespoon extra virgin olive oil; fresh lemon juice to taste)

♦ Sliced pear

♦ 8 ounces green or white tea or spring water

Supplements:

♦ 1 packet of Weight Management supplements

♦ 1 1,000 mg fish oil capsule

♦ 1 astaxanthin capsule

♦ ½ teaspoon glutamine powder—mix in water and drink immediately

BEDTIME:

♦ ½ cup yogurt with 1 tablespoon POM Wonderful pomegranate juice or pure açaí pulp

♦ 4 almonds

♦ 1 peach

♦ 8 ounces spring water

* All recipes can be found in *The Perricone Weight-Loss Diet*

JOURNAL NOTES

THREE THINGS TO CELEBRATE FROM MY DAY:

1. _____

2. _____

3. _____

RECORD THE POSITIVE CHANGES
YOUR BODY EXPERIENCES EACH DAY

Weight: _____   Tone: _____

Energy: _____

Exercise: _____

RECORD THE POSITIVE MENTAL AND
EMOTIONAL EXPERIENCES EACH DAY

Changes in mood: _____

Stress handling: _____

Memory: _____

Problem-solving ability: _____

EMBRACING THE ANTI-INFLAMMATORY LIFESTYLE

Progress in overcoming bad habits:

_____

Progress in minimizing stress:

_____

Cups of coffee: _____   Alcohol: _____

Smoking: _____   Conflict/Tension: _____

Sleep (# of hours): _____   Sleep quality: _____

BENEFITS OF THE GIFT OF QUIET CONTEMPLATION

_____

_____

_____

_____

_____

_____

_____

_____

> Laughter is an excellent antidote to stress—it can lower levels of stress hormones, boost the immune system, and increase feelings of well being.

WEEK 4 / DAY 27   DATE: _____

BREAKFAST:

- 2 egg omelette with ½ ounce feta cheese, 3 cherry tomatoes, halved, and 1 teaspoon chopped green onion
- 2 links turkey sausage
- ½ cup blueberries
- 3 almonds
- 8 ounces spring water

Supplements:

- 1 packet of Weight Management supplements
- 1 1,000 mg fish oil capsule
- 1 astaxanthin capsule
- ½ teaspoon glutamine powder—mix in water and drink immediately

LUNCH:

- **Caribbean Fish Burger*** over baby greens
- ½ cup sliced tomatoes
- ¼ cup **Edamame Guacamole*** or ¼ sliced avocado
- ½ cup black raspberries
- 8 ounces iced green or white tea or spring water

Supplements:

- 1 packet of Weight Management supplements
- 1 1,000 mg fish oil capsule
- 1 astaxanthin capsule
- ½ teaspoon glutamine powder—mix in water and drink immediately

* All recipes can be found in *The Perricone Weight-Loss Diet*

> Studies show that green tea prevents the absorption of fat, helping to keep excess body fat under control.

SNACK:

- 1 ounce sliced turkey
- 2 flax crackers
- 2-inch slice honeydew
- 8 ounces spring water

DINNER:

- Salmon/fish **Mole with Pumpkin and Sunflower Seeds***
- Steamed artichoke
- 1 cup of salad (dark green leafy lettuce, dressed with 1 tablespoon extra virgin olive oil; fresh lemon juice to taste)
- 1 apple
- 8 ounces green tea or spring water

Supplements:

- 1 packet of Weight Management supplements
- 1 1,000 mg fish oil capsule
- 1 astaxanthin capsule
- ½ teaspoon glutamine powder—mix in water and drink immediately

BEDTIME:

- ½ cup cottage cheese topped with 1 tablespoon sesame seeds
- 1 pear
- 8 ounces spring water

* All recipes can be found in *The Perricone Weight-Loss Diet*

JOURNAL NOTES

THREE THINGS TO CELEBRATE FROM MY DAY:

1. _____

2. _____

3. _____

RECORD THE POSITIVE CHANGES
YOUR BODY EXPERIENCES EACH DAY

Weight: _____   Tone: _____

Energy: _____

Exercise: _____

RECORD THE POSITIVE MENTAL AND
EMOTIONAL EXPERIENCES EACH DAY

Changes in mood: _____

Stress handling: _____

Memory: _____

Problem-solving ability: _____

EMBRACING THE ANTI-INFLAMMATORY LIFESTYLE

Progress in overcoming bad habits:

_____

Progress in minimizing stress:

_____

Cups of coffee: _____   Alcohol: _____

Smoking: _____   Conflict/Tension: _____

Sleep (# of hours): _____   Sleep quality: _____

BENEFITS OF THE GIFT OF QUIET CONTEMPLATION

_____

_____

_____

_____

_____

_____

_____

_____

> Choose brightly colored fruits and vegetables
> because they are high in antioxidants, nature's
> anti-inflammatories

WEEK 4 / DAY 28   DATE: _____

BREAKFAST:

♦ 2 eggs, scrambled with chopped green onion and bell pepper

♦ 1 ounce lox

♦ ½ cup (measured dry) **Stop the Clock! Cereal*** with 1 teaspoon flax seed and 1 tablespoon sesame seeds

♦ ½ grapefruit

♦ 8 ounces green or white tea with fresh lemon or spring water

Supplements:

♦ 1 packet of Weight Management supplements

♦ 1 1,000 mg fish oil capsule

♦ 1 astaxanthin capsule

♦ ½ teaspoon glutamine powder—mix in water and drink immediately

LUNCH:

♦ **Sesame Seed-Encrusted Salmon***

♦ Arugula salad with extra virgin olive oil, fresh lemon juice, 3 sliced olives, and 4 cherry tomatoes

♦ 1 pear

♦ 8 ounces spring water

Supplements:

♦ 1 packet of Weight Management supplements

♦ 1 1,000 mg fish oil capsule

♦ 1 astaxanthin capsule

♦ ½ teaspoon glutamine powder—mix in water and drink immediately

* All recipes can be found in *The Perricone Weight-Loss Diet*

SNACK:

- 1 ounce sliced smoked turkey
- 4 walnuts
- 1 apple
- 8 ounces spring water

DINNER:

- **Spicy Fish Stew***
- Wilted spinach or escarole with fresh lemon juice
- 1 cup of salad (dark green leafy lettuce, dressed with 1 tablespoon extra virgin olive oil; fresh lemon juice to taste)
- ½ cup berries
- 8 ounces spring water

Supplements:

- 1 packet of Weight Management supplements
- 1 1,000 mg fish oil capsule
- 1 astaxanthin capsule
- ½ teaspoon glutamine powder—mix in water and drink immediately

BEDTIME:

- Smoothie with ½ cup kefir, 6 cherries, and 1 tablespoon POM Wonderful pomegranate juice or pure açaí pulp

* All recipes can be found in *The Perricone Weight-Loss Diet*

Remember to cleanse and care for you skin
morning and evening

JOURNAL NOTES

THREE THINGS TO CELEBRATE FROM MY DAY:

1. _____

2. _____

3. _____

RECORD THE POSITIVE CHANGES
YOUR BODY EXPERIENCES EACH DAY

Weight: _____   Tone: _____

Energy: _____

Exercise: _____

RECORD THE POSITIVE MENTAL AND
EMOTIONAL EXPERIENCES EACH DAY

Changes in mood: _____

Stress handling: _____

Memory: _____

Problem-solving ability: _____

EMBRACING THE ANTI-INFLAMMATORY LIFESTYLE

Progress in overcoming bad habits:

_____

Progress in minimizing stress:

_____

Cups of coffee: _____   Alcohol: _____

Smoking: _____   Conflict/Tension: _____

Sleep (# of hours): _____   Sleep quality: _____

BENEFITS OF THE GIFT OF QUIET CONTEMPLATION

_____

_____

_____

_____

_____

_____

_____

_____

> **Always remember to eat the protein first at every meal.**

WEEK 5 / DAY 29   DATE: _____

BREAKFAST:

- 2 poached omega-3 eggs with **Indian Spinach***
- 2 slices turkey bacon
- ½ cup honeydew with 1 teaspoon chopped fresh mint
- 8 ounces green tea with slice of ginger or spring water

Supplements:

- 1 packet of Weight Management supplements
- 1 1,000 mg fish oil capsule
- 1 astaxanthin capsule
- ½ teaspoon glutamine powder—mix in water and drink immediately

LUNCH:

- 1½ cups **African Groundnut Stew***
- 1 cup of salad (dark green leafy lettuce, dressed with 1 tablespoon extra virgin olive oil; fresh lemon juice to taste)
- ⅓ cup berries
- 8 ounces spring water

Supplements:

- 1 packet of Weight Management supplements
- 1 1,000 mg fish oil capsule
- 1 astaxanthin capsule
- ½ teaspoon glutamine powder—mix in water and drink immediately

* All recipes can be found in *The Perricone Weight-Loss Diet*

> Animal fats are pro-inflammatory saturated
> fats, so use them in moderation.

SNACK:

- ¼ cup **Edamame Guacamole*** + 1 teaspoon flaxseed served with celery and jicama sticks
- 8 ounces spring water

DINNER:

- Poached or grilled salmon (6–8 ounces raw weight) with **Spring Roll Salad***
- Steamed asparagus
- 2-inch wedge of cantaloupe
- 8 ounces spring water

Supplements:

- 1 packet of Weight Management supplements
- 1 1,000 mg fish oil capsule
- 1 astaxanthin capsule
- ½ teaspoon glutamine powder—mix in water and drink immediately

BEDTIME:

- ¼ cup plain yogurt with ½ teaspoon vanilla
- 1 teaspoon ground flax
- ¼ cup raspberries
- **Moroccan Mint Tea*** or spring water

* All recipes can be found in *The Perricone Weight-Loss Diet*

JOURNAL NOTES

THREE THINGS TO CELEBRATE FROM MY DAY:

1. _____

2. _____

3. _____

RECORD THE POSITIVE CHANGES
YOUR BODY EXPERIENCES EACH DAY

Weight: _____   Tone: _____

Energy: _____

Exercise: _____

RECORD THE POSITIVE MENTAL AND
EMOTIONAL EXPERIENCES EACH DAY

Changes in mood: _____

Stress handling: _____

Memory: _____

Problem-solving ability: _____

EMBRACING THE ANTI-INFLAMMATORY LIFESTYLE

Progress in overcoming bad habits:

_____

Progress in minimizing stress:

_____

Cups of coffee: _____   Alcohol: _____

Smoking: _____   Conflict/Tension: _____

Sleep (# of hours): _____   Sleep quality: _____

BENEFITS OF THE GIFT OF QUIET CONTEMPLATION

_____

_____

_____

_____

_____

_____

_____

_____

_____

> Every meal or snack must include protein, low-glycemic carbs, and essential fatty acids.

WEEK 5 / DAY 30   DATE: _____

BREAKFAST:

- 2 soft-boiled eggs
- ½ cup (measured dry) **Stop the Clock! Cereal*** with 1 tablespoon POM Wonderful pomegranate juice or pure açaí pulp
- ½ cup plain yogurt with ½ cup diced cantaloupe and 1 teaspoon chopped mint
- 8 ounces green tea or spring water

Supplements:

- 1 packet of Weight Management supplements
- 1 1,000 mg fish oil capsule
- 1 astaxanthin capsule
- ½ teaspoon glutamine powder—mix in water and drink immediately

LUNCH:

- **Icy Gazpacho with Fresh Lime***
- Grilled chicken breast (6 ounces raw weight boneless, skinless)
- 1 cup of salad (dark green leafy lettuce, dressed with 1 tablespoon extra virgin olive oil; fresh lemon juice to taste)
- ½ grapefruit
- 8 ounces iced green tea or spring water

Supplements:

- 1 packet of Weight Management supplements
- 1 1,000 mg fish oil capsule
- 1 astaxanthin capsule
- ½ teaspoon glutamine powder—mix in water and drink immediately

* All recipes can be found in *The Perricone Weight-Loss Diet*

> Omega-3 fatty acids found in fish and fish oil help us burn off calories before they get a chance to be stored as fat.

SNACK:

♦ ⅓ cup cottage cheese with 1 tablespoon ground flax and ¼ cup blueberries

♦ 8 ounces spring water

DINNER:

♦ Poached or baked halibut (or salmon) (6–8 ounces raw weight boneless) with **Curried Cabbage***

♦ 1 cup of cherry tomato salad with 1 teaspoon each chopped ginger, cilantro, extra virgin olive oil; low-sodium soy sauce and fresh lemon juice to taste

♦ 1 pear

♦ 8 ounces spring water with fresh lime

Supplements:

♦ 1 packet of Weight Management supplements

♦ 1 1,000 mg fish oil capsule

♦ 1 astaxanthin capsule

♦ ½ teaspoon glutamine powder—mix in water and drink immediately

BEDTIME:

♦ ½ cup kefir

♦ 3 almonds

♦ 6 cherries

♦ 8 ounces spring water

* All recipes can be found in *The Perricone Weight-Loss Diet*

JOURNAL NOTES

THREE THINGS TO CELEBRATE FROM MY DAY:

1. _____

2. _____

3. _____

RECORD THE POSITIVE CHANGES
YOUR BODY EXPERIENCES EACH DAY

Weight: _____   Tone: _____

Energy: _____

Exercise: _____

RECORD THE POSITIVE MENTAL AND
EMOTIONAL EXPERIENCES EACH DAY

Changes in mood: _____

Stress handling: _____

Memory: _____

Problem-solving ability: _____

EMBRACING THE ANTI-INFLAMMATORY LIFESTYLE

Progress in overcoming bad habits:

_____

Progress in minimizing stress:

_____

Cups of coffee: _____   Alcohol: _____

Smoking: _____   Conflict/Tension: _____

Sleep (# of hours): _____   Sleep quality: _____

BENEFITS OF THE GIFT OF QUIET CONTEMPLATION

_____

_____

_____

_____

_____

_____

_____

_____

_____

> **Always eat your protein first.**
> **This will help suppress your appetite.**

WEEK 5 / DAY 31

DATE: _____

BREAKFAST:

- 2 whole eggs plus two egg whites scrambled with 1 slice turkey bacon and **Nutty Tomato Pesto***
- ½ grapefruit
- 8 ounces green tea or spring water

Supplements:

- 1 packet of Weight Management supplements
- 1 1,000 mg fish oil capsule
- 1 astaxanthin capsule
- ½ teaspoon glutamine powder—mix in water and drink immediately

LUNCH:

- Salmon fillet, baked or grilled (4–6 ounces raw weight boneless) with 1 cup **Caponata*** salad served on mixed baby greens
- ½ cup raspberries
- 8 ounces iced white or green tea or spring water

Supplements:

- 1 packet of Weight Management supplements
- 1 1,000 mg fish oil capsule
- 1 astaxanthin capsule
- ½ teaspoon glutamine powder—mix in water and drink immediately

* All recipes can be found in *The Perricone Weight-Loss Diet*

> A good night's sleep can help you wake refreshed, looking radiant and youthful. And, after a good night's sleep, doesn't the world look better, too?

SNACK:

- Smoothie with ½ cup kefir, 1 teaspoon ground flax, and ½ cup sliced strawberries
- 8 ounces spring water

DINNER:

- Grilled shrimp (6 ounces raw weight)
- **Scalloped Tomatoes with Caramelized Onions***
- 1 cup of salad (dark green leafy lettuce, dressed with 1 tablespoon extra virgin olive oil; fresh lemon juice to taste)
- 1 apple
- 8 ounces spring water

Supplements:

- 1 packet of Weight Management supplements
- 1 1,000 mg fish oil capsule
- 1 astaxanthin capsule
- ½ teaspoon glutamine powder—mix in water and drink immediately

BEDTIME:

- 1 ounce sliced smoked salmon with 2 flax crackers
- 1 kiwi
- 8 ounces spring water

* All recipes can be found in *The Perricone Weight-Loss Diet*

JOURNAL NOTES

THREE THINGS TO CELEBRATE FROM MY DAY:

1. _____

2. _____

3. _____

RECORD THE POSITIVE CHANGES
YOUR BODY EXPERIENCES EACH DAY

Weight: _____   Tone: _____

Energy: _____

Exercise: _____

RECORD THE POSITIVE MENTAL AND
EMOTIONAL EXPERIENCES EACH DAY

Changes in mood: _____

Stress handling: _____

Memory: _____

Problem-solving ability: _____

EMBRACING THE ANTI-INFLAMMATORY LIFESTYLE

Progress in overcoming bad habits:

_____

Progress in minimizing stress:

_____

Cups of coffee: _____   Alcohol: _____

Smoking: _____   Conflict/Tension: _____

Sleep (# of hours): _____   Sleep quality: _____

BENEFITS OF THE GIFT OF QUIET CONTEMPLATION

_____

_____

_____

_____

_____

_____

_____

_____

> **Save the fresh fruit for the end of the meal. This will prevent the natural sugars found in the fruit from causing a spike in blood sugar.**

WEEK 5 / DAY 32   DATE: _____

BREAKFAST:

- 1 boiled egg
- ½ cup **Stop the Clock! Cereal***
- ½ cup **Blueberry Compote*** with 1 cup plain yogurt
- 8 ounces green or white tea or spring water

Supplements:

- 1 packet of Weight Management supplements
- 1 1,000 mg fish oil capsule
- 1 astaxanthin capsule
- ½ teaspoon glutamine powder—mix in water and drink immediately

LUNCH:

- Grilled turkey burger (4–6 ounces raw weight) served on baby spinach
- Tossed green salad with ¼ avocado slice
- 1 apple
- 8 ounces iced green tea with lemon or spring water

Supplements:

- 1 packet of Weight Management supplements
- 1 1,000 mg fish oil capsule
- 1 astaxanthin capsule
- ½ teaspoon glutamine powder—mix in water and drink immediately

* All recipes can be found in *The Perricone Weight-Loss Diet*

> Essential fatty acids found in fish and fish oil lower insulin levels. High levels of insulin cause weight gain and block weight loss.

SNACK:

- Cantaloupe wedge wrapped with 1 ounce slice of turkey breast, drizzled with 1 teaspoon flax oil
- 8 ounces spring water

DINNER:

- Grilled salmon (6–8 ounces raw weight) with **Creamy Onion Sauce with Roasted Garlic and Thyme***
- Steamed artichoke
- 1 cup of salad (dark green leafy lettuce, dressed with 1 tablespoon extra virgin olive oil; fresh lemon juice to taste)
- 8 ounces spring water

Supplements:

- 1 packet of Weight Management supplements
- 1 1,000 mg fish oil capsule
- 1 astaxanthin capsule
- ½ teaspoon glutamine powder—mix in water and drink immediately

BEDTIME:

- ¼ cup yogurt mixed with 1 tablespoon POM Wonderful pomegranate juice or pure açaí pulp
- 2 tablespoons sliced almonds
- ½ kiwi, diced
- 8 ounces spring water

* All recipes can be found in *The Perricone Weight-Loss Diet*

JOURNAL NOTES

THREE THINGS TO CELEBRATE FROM MY DAY:

1. _____

2. _____

3. _____

RECORD THE POSITIVE CHANGES
YOUR BODY EXPERIENCES EACH DAY

Weight: _____   Tone: _____

Energy: _____

Exercise: _____

RECORD THE POSITIVE MENTAL AND
EMOTIONAL EXPERIENCES EACH DAY

Changes in mood: _____

Stress handling: _____

Memory: _____

Problem-solving ability: _____

EMBRACING THE ANTI-INFLAMMATORY LIFESTYLE

Progress in overcoming bad habits:

_____

Progress in minimizing stress:

_____

Cups of coffee: _____   Alcohol: _____

Smoking: _____   Conflict/Tension: _____

Sleep (# of hours): _____   Sleep quality: _____

BENEFITS OF THE GIFT OF QUIET CONTEMPLATION

_____

_____

_____

_____

_____

_____

_____

_____

> Looking for a fat-burner, muscle-builder, wrinkle-eraser, skin-saver, depression-lifter, and brain-booster? Try wild Alaskan salmon!

WEEK 5 / DAY 33   DATE: _____

BREAKFAST:

◆ 2 egg omelet with 2 ounces smoked salmon, fresh dill, and cherry tomatoes

◆ ⅓ cup kefir with 2 tablespoons blackberries

◆ 8 ounces green or white tea or spring water

Supplements:

◆ 1 packet of Weight Management supplements

◆ 1 1,000 mg fish oil capsule

◆ 1 astaxanthin capsule

◆ ½ teaspoon glutamine powder—mix in water and drink immediately

LUNCH:

◆ 6 ounces **Egyptian Chicken Salad***

◆ 1 cup **Broccoli Dill Soup with Lemon and Tahini***

◆ 1 apple

◆ 8 ounces spring water

Supplements:

◆ 1 packet of Weight Management supplements

◆ 1 1,000 mg fish oil capsule

◆ 1 astaxanthin capsule

◆ ½ teaspoon glutamine powder—mix in water and drink immediately

* All recipes can be found in *The Perricone Weight-Loss Diet*

> Our goal is to avoid spikes in blood sugar
> because they trigger insulin release.
> Remember this fact: insulin release = stored fat!

SNACK:

- ½ cup yogurt with 1 tablespoon chopped hazelnuts and ¼ cup diced kiwi
- 8 ounces spring water

DINNER:

- Grilled sablefish (or salmon) (6–8 ounces raw weight skinless)
- **Cucumber-Tomato Salad***
- **Brussels Sprouts with Slivered Almonds***
- 8 ounces spring water

Supplements:

- 1 packet of Weight Management supplements
- 1 1,000 mg fish oil capsule
- 1 astaxanthin capsule
- ½ teaspoon glutamine powder—mix in water and drink immediately

BEDTIME:

- ½ cup cottage cheese with 1 teaspoon ground flaxseed and ⅓ cup sliced strawberries
- 8 ounces spring water

* All recipes can be found in *The Perricone Weight-Loss Diet*

JOURNAL NOTES

THREE THINGS TO CELEBRATE FROM MY DAY:

1. _____

2. _____

3. _____

RECORD THE POSITIVE CHANGES
YOUR BODY EXPERIENCES EACH DAY

Weight: _____   Tone: _____

Energy: _____

Exercise: _____

RECORD THE POSITIVE MENTAL AND
EMOTIONAL EXPERIENCES EACH DAY

Changes in mood: _____

Stress handling: _____

Memory: _____

Problem-solving ability: _____

EMBRACING THE ANTI-INFLAMMATORY LIFESTYLE

Progress in overcoming bad habits:

_____

Progress in minimizing stress:

_____

Cups of coffee: _____   Alcohol: _____

Smoking: _____   Conflict/Tension: _____

Sleep (# of hours): _____   Sleep quality: _____

BENEFITS OF THE GIFT OF QUIET CONTEMPLATION

_____

_____

_____

_____

_____

_____

_____

_____

_____

> **If you don't drink water,
> your body cannot metabolize fat.**

WEEK 5 / DAY 34   DATE: _____

BREAKFAST:

- 2 hard-boiled omega-3 eggs
- ½ cup (measured dry) **Stop the Clock! Cereal***
- ⅓ cup blueberries or blackberries plus ¼ cup plain yogurt
- 8 ounces green tea with lemon or spring water

Supplements:

- 1 packet of Weight Management supplements
- 1 1,000 mg fish oil capsule
- 1 astaxanthin capsule
- ½ teaspoon glutamine powder—mix in water and drink immediately

LUNCH:

- Poached or baked salmon (4–6 ounces raw weight boneless)
- 1 cup **Persian Vegetable Soup***
- 1 2-inch wedge honeydew
- 8 ounces spring water

Supplements:

- 1 packet of Weight Management supplements
- 1 1,000 mg fish oil capsule
- 1 astaxanthin capsule
- ½ teaspoon glutamine powder—mix in water and drink immediately

* All recipes can be found in *The Perricone Weight-Loss Diet*

> Eat raw foods for enzymes. Enzymes are critical to good health as they assist in the digestion and absorption of nutrients from food.

SNACK:

- Smoothie with ½ cup kefir, 1 teaspoon flax oil, pinch of cinnamon, and 2 tablespoons raspberries
- 8 ounces spring water

DINNER:

- **Grilled Miso Salmon (or Chicken)*** (6–8 ounces raw weight)
- Sautéed spinach (or escarole) and mushrooms
- 1 cup of salad (dark green leafy lettuce, dressed with 1 tablespoon extra virgin olive oil; fresh lemon juice to taste)
- 1 apple
- 8 ounces green tea or spring water

Supplements:

- 1 packet of Weight Management supplements
- 1 1,000 mg fish oil capsule
- 1 astaxanthin capsule
- ½ teaspoon glutamine powder—mix in water and drink immediately

BEDTIME:

- 1 ounce slice smoked chicken
- 4 walnuts
- 1 2-inch wedge honeydew
- 8 ounces spring water

* All recipes can be found in *The Perricone Weight-Loss Diet*

JOURNAL NOTES

THREE THINGS TO CELEBRATE FROM MY DAY:

1. _____

2. _____

3. _____

RECORD THE POSITIVE CHANGES
YOUR BODY EXPERIENCES EACH DAY

Weight: _____   Tone: _____

Energy: _____

Exercise: _____

RECORD THE POSITIVE MENTAL AND
EMOTIONAL EXPERIENCES EACH DAY

Changes in mood: _____

Stress handling: _____

Memory: _____

Problem-solving ability: _____

EMBRACING THE ANTI-INFLAMMATORY LIFESTYLE

Progress in overcoming bad habits:

_____

Progress in minimizing stress:

_____

Cups of coffee: _____   Alcohol: _____

Smoking: _____   Conflict/Tension: _____

Sleep (# of hours): _____   Sleep quality: _____

BENEFITS OF THE GIFT OF QUIET CONTEMPLATION

_____

_____

_____

_____

_____

_____

_____

_____

> Enzyme-rich sprouted seeds are tiny power-houses of anti-inflammatory antioxidants and an outstanding source of many nutrients.

WEEK 5 / DAY 35

DATE: _____

BREAKFAST:

- 2 ounces lox
- 2 flax crackers
- 2 soft-boiled eggs
- ½ grapefruit
- 8 ounces green tea with lemon or spring water

Supplements:

- 1 packet of Weight Management supplements
- 1 1,000 mg fish oil capsule
- 1 astaxanthin capsule
- ½ teaspoon glutamine powder—mix in water and drink immediately

LUNCH:

- **Egyptian Chicken Salad***
- 1 apple
- 8 ounces spring water

Supplements:

- 1 packet of Weight Management supplements
- 1 1,000 mg fish oil capsule
- 1 astaxanthin capsule
- ½ teaspoon glutamine powder—mix in water and drink immediately

* All recipes can be found in *The Perricone Weight-Loss Diet*

Adding fiber to the diet helps regulate blood sugar levels, important in avoiding diabetes, metabolic disorders, and unwanted weight gain.

SNACK:

♦ ½ cup plain yogurt topped with 1 tablespoon POM Wonderful pomegranate juice or pure açaí pulp

♦ 2 tablespoons sesame seeds

♦ ⅓ cup blueberries

♦ 8 ounces spring water

DINNER:

♦ **Pan-Roasted Salmon with Wilted Chard and Tomato-Mint Raita***

♦ 1 cup of salad (dark green leafy lettuce, dressed with 1 tablespoon extra virgin olive oil; fresh lemon juice to taste)

♦ 1 pear

♦ 8 ounces white or green tea with lemon, or spring water

Supplements:

♦ 1 packet of Weight Management supplements

♦ 1 1,000 mg fish oil capsule

♦ 1 astaxanthin capsule

♦ ½ teaspoon glutamine powder—mix in water and drink immediately

BEDTIME:

♦ ½ cup cottage cheese with 1 diced apple and 4 slivered almonds

♦ 8 ounces spring water

* All recipes can be found in *The Perricone Weight-Loss Diet*

JOURNAL NOTES

THREE THINGS TO CELEBRATE FROM MY DAY:

1. _____

2. _____

3. _____

RECORD THE POSITIVE CHANGES
YOUR BODY EXPERIENCES EACH DAY

Weight: _____   Tone: _____

Energy: _____

Exercise: _____

RECORD THE POSITIVE MENTAL AND
EMOTIONAL EXPERIENCES EACH DAY

Changes in mood: _____

Stress handling: _____

Memory: _____

Problem-solving ability: _____

EMBRACING THE ANTI-INFLAMMATORY LIFESTYLE

Progress in overcoming bad habits:

_____

Progress in minimizing stress:

_____

Cups of coffee: _____   Alcohol: _____

Smoking: _____   Conflict/Tension: _____

Sleep (# of hours): _____   Sleep quality: _____

BENEFITS OF THE GIFT OF QUIET CONTEMPLATION

_____

_____

_____

_____

_____

_____

_____

_____

_____

> Eat the skins of your fruits and vegetables if they are organic and unwaxed; the most fiber and greatest antioxidant/anti-inflammatory properties are in the skin.

WEEK 6 / DAY 36   DATE: _____

BREAKFAST:

- ½ cup cooked old-fashioned oatmeal, topped with 2 tablespoons yogurt, ¼ cup blueberries and 2 tablespoons sesame seeds
- 3 slices soy or turkey bacon
- 8 ounces green tea or spring water

Supplements:

- 1 packet of Weight Management supplements
- 1 1,000 mg fish oil capsule
- 1 astaxanthin capsule
- ½ teaspoon glutamine powder—mix in water and drink immediately

LUNCH:

- Halibut or salmon fillet, grilled, poached, or steamed (4–6 ounces raw weight boneless)
- **Miso Soup with Wilted Greens and Roasted Tomatoes***
- 1 pear
- 8 ounces green tea or spring water

Supplements:

- 1 packet of Weight Management supplements
- 1 1,000 mg fish oil capsule
- 1 astaxanthin capsule
- ½ teaspoon glutamine powder—mix in water and drink immediately

* All recipes can be found in *The Perricone Weight-Loss Diet*

> Fats with anti-inflammatory action are mono or polyunsaturated, and include extra virgin olive oil and foods rich in essential fatty acids (salmon, coconut, avocados, açaí, olives, nuts and seeds).

SNACK:

- ½ cup cottage cheese with 2 tablespoons salsa and 2 teaspoons sesame seeds
- 8 ounces spring water

DINNER:

- **Curried Stew*** with chicken, turkey, or tofu
- 1 cup of salad (dark green leafy lettuce, dressed with 1 tablespoon extra virgin olive oil; fresh lemon juice to taste)
- ½ cup mixed berries
- 8 ounces spring water

Supplements:

- 1 packet of Weight Management supplements
- 1 1,000 mg fish oil capsule
- 1 astaxanthin capsule
- ½ teaspoon glutamine powder—mix in water and drink immediately

BEDTIME:

- 1 hard-boiled egg
- Celery sticks and 2 tablespoons hummus
- 8 ounces spring water

* All recipes can be found in *The Perricone Weight-Loss Diet*

JOURNAL NOTES

THREE THINGS TO CELEBRATE FROM MY DAY:

1. _____

2. _____

3. _____

RECORD THE POSITIVE CHANGES
YOUR BODY EXPERIENCES EACH DAY

Weight: _____   Tone: _____

Energy: _____

Exercise: _____

RECORD THE POSITIVE MENTAL AND
EMOTIONAL EXPERIENCES EACH DAY

Changes in mood: _____

Stress handling: _____

Memory: _____

Problem-solving ability: _____

EMBRACING THE ANTI-INFLAMMATORY LIFESTYLE

Progress in overcoming bad habits:

_____

Progress in minimizing stress:

_____

Cups of coffee: _____   Alcohol: _____

Smoking: _____   Conflict/Tension: _____

Sleep (# of hours): _____   Sleep quality: _____

BENEFITS OF THE GIFT OF QUIET CONTEMPLATION

_____

_____

_____

_____

_____

_____

_____

_____

> A simple rule of thumb is to consider the following: if it contains flour, and/or sugar or other sweetener it will be pro-inflammatory.

WEEK 6 / DAY 37   DATE: _____

BREAKFAST:

- 2 whole eggs plus 1 egg white omelet with 3 tablespoons **Baba Ghanouj***
- 6 cherry tomatoes, halved and 1 teaspoon chopped cilantro
- ¾ cup plain yogurt with 2 tablespoons chopped almonds and ¼ teaspoon pure vanilla extract
- ½ grapefruit
- 8 ounces white or green tea or spring water

Supplements:

- 1 packet of Weight Management supplements
- 1 1,000 mg fish oil capsule
- 1 astaxanthin capsule
- ½ teaspoon glutamine powder—mix in water and drink immediately

LUNCH:

- **Tomato Avocado Soup with Fresh Crabmeat***
- 1 cup of salad (dark green leafy lettuce, dressed with 1 tablespoon extra virgin olive oil; fresh lemon juice to taste)
- ½ cup black raspberries
- 8 ounces iced green tea with lemon, or spring water

Supplements:

- 1 packet of Weight Management supplements
- 1 1,000 mg fish oil capsule
- 1 astaxanthin capsule
- ½ teaspoon glutamine powder—mix in water and drink immediately

* All recipes can be found in *The Perricone Weight-Loss Diet*

> An apple a day . . . a recent study showed that eating three small apples or pears per day appears to accelerate weight loss in women.

SNACK:

♦ Smoothie with ½ cup kefir, ¼ cup almond milk, and 6 (pitted) cherries

♦ 8 ounces spring water

DINNER:

♦ Grilled chicken (or salmon) (6–9 ounces raw weight boneless skinless) with **Pomegranate Walnut Sauce***

♦ Steamed kale

♦ 1 sliced pear

♦ 8 ounces **Moroccan Mint Tea*** or spring water

Supplements:

♦ 1 packet of Weight Management supplements

♦ 1 1,000 mg fish oil capsule

♦ 1 astaxanthin capsule

♦ ½ teaspoon glutamine powder—mix in water and drink immediately

BEDTIME:

♦ 2 ounces thinly sliced turkey breast

♦ 4 almonds

♦ 1 2-inch wedge honeydew

♦ 8 ounces spring water

* All recipes can be found in *The Perricone Weight-Loss Diet*

JOURNAL NOTES

THREE THINGS TO CELEBRATE FROM MY DAY:

1. _____

2. _____

3. _____

RECORD THE POSITIVE CHANGES
YOUR BODY EXPERIENCES EACH DAY

Weight: _____   Tone: _____

Energy: _____

Exercise: _____

RECORD THE POSITIVE MENTAL AND
EMOTIONAL EXPERIENCES EACH DAY

Changes in mood: _____

Stress handling: _____

Memory: _____

Problem-solving ability: _____

EMBRACING THE ANTI-INFLAMMATORY LIFESTYLE

Progress in overcoming bad habits:

_____

Progress in minimizing stress:

_____

Cups of coffee: _____   Alcohol: _____

Smoking: _____   Conflict/Tension: _____

Sleep (# of hours): _____   Sleep quality: _____

BENEFITS OF THE GIFT OF QUIET CONTEMPLATION

_____

_____

_____

_____

_____

_____

_____

_____

_____

> Try sugar-free salsa. Salsas contain hot peppers whose active ingredient, capsaicin, speeds up the body's metabolism and stimulates the production of saliva, which stimulates the digestive process.

WEEK 6 / DAY 38   DATE: _____

BREAKFAST:

- ◆ 3 egg omelet made with 2 egg whites, 1 whole egg, ¼ cup chopped roasted bell pepper, 2 tablespoons sautéed red onion and 1 teaspoon chopped basil
- ◆ ½ cup (measured dry) **Stop the Clock! Cereal*** cooked with water and ½ teaspoon ground cinnamon
- ◆ ½ cup fresh blueberries
- ◆ 8 ounces green tea or spring water

Supplements:

- ◆ 1 packet of Weight Management supplements
- ◆ 1 1,000 mg fish oil capsule
- ◆ 1 astaxanthin capsule
- ◆ ½ teaspoon glutamine powder—mix in water and drink immediately

LUNCH:

- ◆ **Asian Salad*** with 6 ounces grilled tofu or chicken breast
- ◆ ½ grapefruit
- ◆ 8 ounces iced green tea with lemon, or spring water

Supplements:

- ◆ 1 packet of Weight Management supplements
- ◆ 1 1,000 mg fish oil capsule
- ◆ 1 astaxanthin capsule
- ◆ ½ teaspoon glutamine powder—mix in water and drink immediately

* All recipes can be found in *The Perricone Weight-Loss Diet*

> **Anti-inflammatory foods encourage the burning of fat for energy, eliminate food cravings, and do not stimulate the appetite.**

SNACK:

- ½ cup plain yogurt with 1 tablespoon sesame seeds and 1 tablespoon pure açaí pulp or POM Wonderful pomegranate juice
- 8 ounces spring water

DINNER:

- **Three-Fish Etouffée with Baby Artichokes and Spicy Tomato Broth***
- 1 cup of salad (dark green leafy lettuce, dressed with 1 tablespoon extra virgin olive oil; fresh lemon juice to taste)
- 1 apple
- 8 ounces white tea with ginger slice, or spring water

Supplements:

- 1 packet of Weight Management supplements
- 1 1,000 mg fish oil capsule
- 1 astaxanthin capsule
- ½ teaspoon glutamine powder—mix in water and drink immediately

BEDTIME:

- Smoothie with ½ cup kefir, 2 tablespoons blackberries and 1 tablespoon POM Wonderful pomegranate juice or pure açaí pulp
- 8 ounces spring water

* All recipes can be found in *The Perricone Weight-Loss Diet*

JOURNAL NOTES

THREE THINGS TO CELEBRATE FROM MY DAY:

1. _____

2. _____

3. _____

RECORD THE POSITIVE CHANGES
YOUR BODY EXPERIENCES EACH DAY

Weight: _____   Tone: _____

Energy: _____

Exercise: _____

RECORD THE POSITIVE MENTAL AND
EMOTIONAL EXPERIENCES EACH DAY

Changes in mood: _____

Stress handling: _____

Memory: _____

Problem-solving ability: _____

EMBRACING THE ANTI-INFLAMMATORY LIFESTYLE

Progress in overcoming bad habits:

_____

Progress in minimizing stress:

_____

Cups of coffee: _____   Alcohol: _____

Smoking: _____   Conflict/Tension: _____

Sleep (# of hours): _____   Sleep quality: _____

BENEFITS OF THE GIFT OF QUIET CONTEMPLATION

_____

_____

_____

_____

_____

_____

_____

_____

_____

> **Add some sesame seeds to your salad—studies show they promote fat burning.**

WEEK 6 / DAY 39　　　　　　　　　DATE: _____

BREAKFAST:

- 2 eggs scrambled with 2 ounces sliced smoked salmon and 1 teaspoon chopped chives
- ¼ cup (measured dry) **Stop the Clock! Cereal*** with ¼ teaspoon ground ginger
- ½ cup sliced strawberries
- 8 ounces green tea or spring water

Supplements:

- 1 packet of Weight Management supplements
- 1 1,000 mg fish oil capsule
- 1 astaxanthin capsule
- ½ teaspoon glutamine powder—mix in water and drink immediately

LUNCH:

- Grilled sesame tofu or chicken (6 ounces)
- **Tomato-Ginger Bisque***
- 1 sliced kiwi
- 8 ounces spring water

Supplements:

- 1 packet of Weight Management supplements
- 1 1,000 mg fish oil capsule
- 1 astaxanthin capsule
- ½ teaspoon glutamine powder—mix in water and drink immediately

* All recipes can be found in *The Perricone Weight-Loss Diet*

> Exercise not only helps us to lose weight and gain muscle, it is also proven as a stress reducer and mood elevator.

SNACK:

- ♦ ½ cup cottage cheese with 1 teaspoon flaxseed and ⅓ cup diced apple
- ♦ 8 ounces spring water

DINNER:

- ♦ **Salmon Chermoula***
- ♦ 1 cup of salad (dark green leafy lettuce, dressed with 1 tablespoon extra virgin olive oil; fresh lemon juice to taste)
- ♦ 1 cup steamed broccoli
- ♦ 1 Asian pear
- ♦ 8 ounces spring water

Supplements:

- ♦ 1 packet of Weight Management supplements
- ♦ 1 1,000 mg fish oil capsule
- ♦ 1 astaxanthin capsule
- ♦ ½ teaspoon glutamine powder—mix in water and drink immediately

BEDTIME:

- ♦ 1 ounce sliced turkey
- ♦ ¼ avocado
- ♦ 8 ounces spring water

* All recipes can be found in *The Perricone Weight-Loss Diet*

JOURNAL NOTES

THREE THINGS TO CELEBRATE FROM MY DAY:

1. _____

2. _____

3. _____

RECORD THE POSITIVE CHANGES
YOUR BODY EXPERIENCES EACH DAY

Weight: _____   Tone: _____

Energy: _____

Exercise: _____

RECORD THE POSITIVE MENTAL AND
EMOTIONAL EXPERIENCES EACH DAY

Changes in mood: _____

Stress handling: _____

Memory: _____

Problem-solving ability: _____

EMBRACING THE ANTI-INFLAMMATORY LIFESTYLE

Progress in overcoming bad habits:

_____

Progress in minimizing stress:

_____

Cups of coffee: _____   Alcohol: _____

Smoking: _____   Conflict/Tension: _____

Sleep (# of hours): _____   Sleep quality: _____

BENEFITS OF THE GIFT OF QUIET CONTEMPLATION

_____

_____

_____

_____

_____

_____

_____

_____

> **Find ways to minimize stress because it promotes weight gain.**

WEEK 6 / DAY 40　　　　　DATE: _____

BREAKFAST:

- ◆ Grilled salmon fillet (4 ounces raw weight boneless)
- ◆ 6 cherry tomatoes
- ◆ ⅓ cup sliced strawberries
- ◆ 8 ounces green tea or spring water

Supplements:

- ◆ 1 packet of Weight Management supplements
- ◆ 1 1,000 mg fish oil capsule
- ◆ 1 astaxanthin capsule
- ◆ ½ teaspoon glutamine powder—mix in water and drink immediately

LUNCH:

- ◆ Grilled chicken breast (6 ounces raw weight boneless skinless) or tofu veggie burger
- ◆ 1 cup **Watercress and Almond Salad with Roasted Onion Dressing***
- ◆ ½ cup cherries
- ◆ 8 ounces spring water

Supplements:

- ◆ 1 packet of Weight Management supplements
- ◆ 1 1,000 mg fish oil capsule
- ◆ 1 astaxanthin capsule
- ◆ ½ teaspoon glutamine powder—mix in water and drink immediately

* All recipes can be found in *The Perricone Weight-Loss Diet*

> **Chronic, high stress levels cause us to overeat and to store fat in the abdominal region.**

SNACK:

- 1 ounce sliced chicken or turkey breast
- 4 almonds
- 1 apple
- 8 ounces spring water

DINNER:

- Salmon, trout, or mackerel (4–6 ounces raw weight boneless) with **Baba Ghanouj***
- Green beans sautéed with garlic and sesame oil
- 1 cup of salad (dark green leafy lettuce, dressed with 1 tablespoon extra virgin olive oil; fresh lemon juice to taste)
- Sliced pear
- 8 ounces green or white tea or spring water

    Supplements:

    - 1 packet of Weight Management supplements
    - 1 1,000 mg fish oil capsule
    - 1 astaxanthin capsule
    - ½ teaspoon glutamine powder—mix in water and drink immediately

BEDTIME:

- ½ cup yogurt with 1 tablespoon POM Wonderful pomegranate juice or pure açaí pulp
- 4 almonds
- 1 peach
- 8 ounces spring water

    * All recipes can be found in *The Perricone Weight-Loss Diet*

JOURNAL NOTES

THREE THINGS TO CELEBRATE FROM MY DAY:

1. _____

2. _____

3. _____

RECORD THE POSITIVE CHANGES
YOUR BODY EXPERIENCES EACH DAY

Weight: _____   Tone: _____

Energy: _____

Exercise: _____

RECORD THE POSITIVE MENTAL AND
EMOTIONAL EXPERIENCES EACH DAY

Changes in mood: _____

Stress handling: _____

Memory: _____

Problem-solving ability: _____

EMBRACING THE ANTI-INFLAMMATORY LIFESTYLE

Progress in overcoming bad habits:

_____

Progress in minimizing stress:

_____

Cups of coffee: _____   Alcohol: _____

Smoking: _____   Conflict/Tension: _____

Sleep (# of hours): _____   Sleep quality: _____

BENEFITS OF THE GIFT OF QUIET CONTEMPLATION

_____

_____

_____

_____

_____

_____

_____

_____

_____

> Laughter is an excellent antidote to stress—it can lower levels of stress hormones, boost the immune system, and increase feelings of well being.

WEEK 6 / DAY 41   DATE: _____

BREAKFAST:

- 2 egg omelette with ½ ounce feta cheese, 3 cherry tomatoes, halved, and 1 teaspoon chopped green onion
- 2 links turkey sausage
- ½ cup blueberries
- 3 almonds
- 8 ounces spring water

Supplements:

- 1 packet of Weight Management supplements
- 1 1,000 mg fish oil capsule
- 1 astaxanthin capsule
- ½ teaspoon glutamine powder—mix in water and drink immediately

LUNCH:

- **Caribbean Fish Burger*** over baby greens
- ½ cup sliced tomatoes
- ¼ cup **Edamame Guacamole*** or ¼ sliced avocado
- ½ cup black raspberries
- 8 ounces iced green or white tea or spring water

Supplements:

- 1 packet of Weight Management supplements
- 1 1,000 mg fish oil capsule
- 1 astaxanthin capsule
- ½ teaspoon glutamine powder—mix in water and drink immediately

* All recipes can be found in *The Perricone Weight-Loss Diet*

SNACK:

- 1 ounce sliced turkey
- 2 flax crackers
- 2-inch slice honeydew
- 8 ounces spring water

DINNER:

- Salmon/fish **Mole with Pumpkin and Sunflower Seeds***
- Steamed artichoke
- 1 cup of salad (dark green leafy lettuce, dressed with 1 tablespoon extra virgin olive oil; fresh lemon juice to taste)
- 1 apple
- 8 ounces green tea or spring water

Supplements:

- 1 packet of Weight Management supplements
- 1 1,000 mg fish oil capsule
- 1 astaxanthin capsule
- ½ teaspoon glutamine powder—mix in water and drink immediately

BEDTIME:

- ½ cup cottage cheese topped with 1 tablespoon sesame seeds
- 1 pear
- 8 ounces spring water

* All recipes can be found in *The Perricone Weight-Loss Diet*

JOURNAL NOTES

THREE THINGS TO CELEBRATE FROM MY DAY:

1. _____

2. _____

3. _____

RECORD THE POSITIVE CHANGES
YOUR BODY EXPERIENCES EACH DAY

Weight: _____   Tone: _____

Energy: _____

Exercise: _____

RECORD THE POSITIVE MENTAL AND
EMOTIONAL EXPERIENCES EACH DAY

Changes in mood: _____

Stress handling: _____

Memory: _____

Problem-solving ability: _____

EMBRACING THE ANTI-INFLAMMATORY LIFESTYLE

Progress in overcoming bad habits:

_____

Progress in minimizing stress:

_____

Cups of coffee: _____   Alcohol: _____

Smoking: _____   Conflict/Tension: _____

Sleep (# of hours): _____   Sleep quality: _____

BENEFITS OF THE GIFT OF QUIET CONTEMPLATION

_____

_____

_____

_____

_____

_____

_____

_____

_____

> Choose brightly colored fruits and vegetables because they are high in antioxidants, nature's anti-inflammatories

WEEK 6 / DAY 42   DATE: _____

BREAKFAST:

- ◆ 2 eggs, scrambled with chopped green onion and bell pepper
- ◆ 1 ounce lox
- ◆ ½ cup (measured dry) **Stop the Clock! Cereal*** with 1 teaspoon flax seed and 1 tablespoon sesame seeds
- ◆ ½ grapefruit
- ◆ 8 ounces green or white tea with fresh lemon or spring water

Supplements:

- ◆ 1 packet of Weight Management supplements
- ◆ 1 1,000 mg fish oil capsule
- ◆ 1 astaxanthin capsule
- ◆ ½ teaspoon glutamine powder—mix in water and drink immediately

LUNCH:

- ◆ **Sesame Seed-Encrusted Salmon***
- ◆ Arugula salad with extra virgin olive oil, fresh lemon juice, 3 sliced olives, and 4 cherry tomatoes
- ◆ 1 pear
- ◆ 8 ounces spring water

Supplements:

- ◆ 1 packet of Weight Management supplements
- ◆ 1 1,000 mg fish oil capsule
- ◆ 1 astaxanthin capsule
- ◆ ½ teaspoon glutamine powder—mix in water and drink immediately

* All recipes can be found in *The Perricone Weight-Loss Diet*

SNACK:

- ◆ 1 ounce sliced smoked turkey
- ◆ 4 walnuts
- ◆ 1 apple
- ◆ 8 ounces spring water

DINNER:

- ◆ **Spicy Fish Stew***
- ◆ Wilted spinach or escarole with fresh lemon juice
- ◆ 1 cup of salad (dark green leafy lettuce, dressed with 1 tablespoon extra virgin olive oil; fresh lemon juice to taste)
- ◆ ½ cup berries
- ◆ 8 ounces spring water

Supplements:

- ◆ 1 packet of Weight Management supplements
- ◆ 1 1,000 mg fish oil capsule
- ◆ 1 astaxanthin capsule
- ◆ ½ teaspoon glutamine powder—mix in water and drink immediately

BEDTIME:

- ◆ Smoothie with ½ cup Kefir, 6 cherries, and 1 tablespoon POM Wonderful pomegranate juice or pure açaí pulp

* All recipes can be found in *The Perricone Weight-Loss Diet*

JOURNAL NOTES

THREE THINGS TO CELEBRATE FROM MY DAY:

1. _____

2. _____

3. _____

RECORD THE POSITIVE CHANGES
YOUR BODY EXPERIENCES EACH DAY

Weight: _____   Tone: _____

Energy: _____

Exercise: _____

RECORD THE POSITIVE MENTAL AND
EMOTIONAL EXPERIENCES EACH DAY

Changes in mood: _____

Stress handling: _____

Memory: _____

Problem-solving ability: _____

EMBRACING THE ANTI-INFLAMMATORY LIFESTYLE

Progress in overcoming bad habits:

_____

Progress in minimizing stress:

_____

Cups of coffee: _____   Alcohol: _____

Smoking: _____   Conflict/Tension: _____

Sleep (# of hours): _____   Sleep quality: _____

BENEFITS OF THE GIFT OF QUIET CONTEMPLATION

_____

_____

_____

_____

_____

_____

_____

_____

_____

RESOURCES

NUTRITIONAL SUPPLEMENTS

Weight Management Supplements

Weight Management Program™ supplements formulated by Dr. Perricone are available at:

♦ N.V. Perricone, M.D., Ltd. at 888-823-7837 or www.nvperriconemd.com

♦ N.V. Perricone, M.D., Ltd. Flagship Store at 791 Madison Avenue (at 67th St.), New York, NY

Anti-aging, Anti-inflammatory Supplements

Skin and Total Body Nutritional Supplements™ formulated by Dr. Perricone are available at:

♦ N.V. Perricone, M.D., Ltd. at 888-823-7837 or www.nvperriconemd.com

♦ N.V. Perricone M.D., Ltd. Flagship Store at 791 Madison Avenue (at 67th St.), New York, NY

♦ All retail partners listed on page 189–190

♦ Optimum Health International (Stephen Sinatra, M.D.) at 800-228-1507 or www.opthealth.com

♦ Life Extension Foundation at 800-544-4440 or www.lef.org

Pure Wild Alaskan Sockeye Salmon Omega-3 Fish Oil

♦ N.V. Perricone, M.D., Ltd. at 888-823-7837 or www.nvperriconemd.com

♦ N.V. Perricone, M.D., Ltd. Flagship Store at 791 Madison Ave (at 67th St.), New York, NY

♦ Optimum Health International (Stephen Sinatra, M.D.) at 800-228-1507 or www.opthealth.com

Glutamine—USP Pharmaceutical-grade Micronized L-glutamine

♦ N.V. Perricone, M.D., Ltd. at 888-823-7837 or www.nvperriconemd.com

Astaxanthin

(highly potent antioxidant found in salmon and marine zooplankton)

♦ N.V. Perricone, M.D., Ltd. at 888-823-7837 or www.nvperriconemd.com
♦ All retail partners listed on page 189–190

Polysaccharide Peptide Food™

This anti-inflammatory, antiaging beverage mix and food topping is custom-manufactured to Dr. Perricone's specifications.

♦ N.V. Perricone, M.D., Ltd. at 888-823-7837 or www.nvperriconemd.com
♦ N.V. Perricone, M.D., Ltd. Flagship Store at 791 Madison Avenue (at 67th St.), New York, NY
♦ All retail partners listed on page 189–190

Maitake D-Fraction® and SX-Fraction® Extract

♦ N.V. Perricone, M.D., Ltd. at 888-823-7837 or www.nvperriconemd.com
♦ Maitake Products, Inc. at 800-747-7418 or www.maitake.com
♦ All retail partners listed on page 189–190

For more information, you may read Maitake Magic (Freedom Press) by Harry Preuss, M.D., available on www.amazon.com and independent bookstores.

Benfotiamine (Anti-Glycation Supplement)

♦ N.V. Perricone, M.D., Ltd. at 888-823-7837 or www.nvperriconemd.com

Anti-inflammatory herbal supplements

New Chapter, Inc. markets potent anti-inflammatory herbal extracts. The company employs CO_2, water, and alcohol extraction to yield an unusually broad spectrum of active constituents from ginger, turmeric, rosemary, and other anti-inflammatory herbs.

♦ www.new-chapter.com or 800-543-7279

DR. PERRICONE'S SUPER FOODS

Wild Alaskan Salmon and Seafood; Wild Organic Berries

Vital Choice Seafood offers wild-harvested fresh-frozen fish (salmon, sablefish, sardines, tuna, and halibut) and fresh-frozen organic blueberries, raspberries and strawberries. Their fish are flash-frozen on the boats and packed in dry ice for delivery via Federal Express or UPS. Compared with farmed salmon, wild Alaskan salmon offers greater purity and a healthier fatty acid profile (less saturated fat and a higher ratio of omega-3 fatty acids to omega-6 fatty acids).

♦ www.vitalchoice.com or 800-608-4825

Açaí (Amazonian Fruit High in Antioxidants)

Açaí fruit has more antioxidants than wild blueberries, pomegranates, or red wine; it also contains essential omega-3s fatty acids, amino acids, calcium, and fiber. Bossa Nova brand açaí is available in grocery, natural supermarkets, and specialty stores across the country.

♦ www.bossausa.com

Avocados

The California Avocado Board offers recipes and health information at www.avocado.org and www.spectrumorganics.com

Beans and lentils (Organic and Heirloom)

♦ Bob's Red Mill sells direct at www.bobsredmill.com or 800-349-2173.
♦ Diamond Organics, Inc., sells direct at www.diamondorganics.com or 888-674-2642.
♦ Westbrae Natural sells through retailers. For locations, go to www.westbrae.com/products/index.html or call 800-434-4246.

Chili peppers

♦ Whole Foods Market (www.wholefoods.com) or Wild Oats (www.wildoats.com)
♦ Diamond Organics, Inc., at www.diamondorganics.com or 888-674-2642

Grain-Free Crackers

♦ Foods Alive Organic Golden Flax Crackers at www.foodsalive.com

Flaxseed

♦ Bob's Red Mill at www.bobsredmill.com or 800-349-2173

Grains

♦ Bob's Red Mill sells a full selection, including whole organic buckwheat and oats online at www.bobsredmill.com or 800-349-2173.

Grass-Fed and Organic Meats

Eatwild.com is an information clearinghouse for consumers seeking grass-fed and organic beef, lamb, goat, bison, poultry, and dairy products. The site's principal researcher and writer is Jo Robinson, the *New York Times* bestselling author of *Pasture Perfect* and *The Omega Diet* (written with renowned fatty acid researcher Dr. Artemis Simopoulos).

♦ www.eatwild.com

Kefir and yogurt

♦ Helios Nutrition is a small organic dairy in Sauk Centre, Minnesota, that makes several flavors of organic kefir with added FOS (prebiotic polysaccharide). Locate retail outlets at 888-3 HELIOS or www.heliosnutrition.com/html/where_to_buy.html

♦ Lifeway Foods of Morton Grove, Illinois, makes kefir and related products with national distribution. Go to www.lifeway.net

♦ Stonyfield Farm Yogurt (natural and organic varieties) is available at many food markets. See the store locator at www.stonyfield.com/StoreLocator/.

♦ Horizon Organic yogurt is available at many food markets. See the store locator at www.horizonorganic/findingproducts/index.html

Luo Han Kuo (Uniquely High in Antioxidants)

♦ N.V. Perricone, M.D., Ltd. at 888-823-7837 or www.nvperriconemd.com

♦ Longjiang River Health Products, LLC, www.LHKHealth.com

Pomegranate Juice and Concentrate (Extremely High in Anti-oxidants)

♦ POM Wonderful is available at 310-966-5800 or www.pomwonderful.com

♦ Also available at supermarkets and natural food stores

Organic Extra Virgin Olive Oil

♦ N.V. Perricone, M.D., Ltd. at 888-823-7837 or www.nvperriconemd.com

♦ N.V. Perricone, M.D., Ltd. Flagship Store at 791 Madison Avenue (at 67th St.), New York, NY

♦ Soler Romero Organic Extra Virgin Olive Oil (superior quality and flavor) available through www.odysseyfoods.com or 360-825-2814

♦ International Olive Oil Council at www.internationaloliveoil.org

♦ California Olive Growers at www.oliveoilsource.com/oliveoildr.htm

Retail outlets (Natural and Organic Foods)

♦ Diamond Organics, Inc., is a direct-to-consumer Internet retailer of certified organic fruits, vegetables, nuts, grains, beans, spices, and more www.diamondorganics.com or 888-674-2642.

♦ Whole Foods Market www.wholefoods.com and Wild Oats www.wildoats.com. These are the two largest natural foods supermarket chains in the United States. Both sell every kind of fresh food (e.g., fish, meat, poultry, fruits, vegetables, eggs, cheese, kefir, yogurt), frozen food, and grocery items (bulk grains, nuts, seeds, beans, cereals, canned goods, sauces, condiments) you would find in a regular supermarket, but without synthetic additives or sweeteners. Their selections include many certified organic foods as well as natural health and body care items. Log onto their websites to find a store near you.

Sprouts: Information and Supplies

♦ The International Sprout Growers Association (ISGA) is the professional association of sprout growers and companies that supply products and services to the sprout industry. Visit their website for outstanding information, recipes, and health notes at www.isga-sprouts.org

- "Sproutman" Steve Meyerowitz is one of the world's leading proponents of do-it-yourself sprouting. 413-528-5200, www.sproutman.com , or P.O. Box 1100, Great Barrington, MA 01230.

Wide Assortment of Teas Including Jasmine/Green Tea
- N.V. Perricone, M.D., Ltd. at 888-823-7837 or www.nvperriconemd.com
- N.V. Perricone, M.D., Ltd. Flagship Store at 791 Madison Avenue (at 67th St.), New York, NY.
- Red Blossom Tea Company at 415-395-0868 or www.redblossomtea.com

Pure Water
- Fiji Water. From the Fiji Islands, this natural artesian water is filtered for centuries through volcanic geology. Available nationwide and at www.fijiwater.com
- Poland Spring Natural Spring Water. Pure and natural spring water from Maine available nation-wide or at www.polandspring.com
- Jana Skinny Water™

Specialty Water
Special Perricone-formulated antiaging water for cellular repair and hydration
- N.V. Perricone, M.D., Ltd. at 888-823-7837 or www.nvperriconemd.com
- N.V. Perricone, M.D., Ltd. Flagship Store at 791 Madison Avenue (at 67th St.), New York, NY

COSMECEUTICAL SKIN CARE

Antioxidant, anti-inflammatory topical products—formulated by Dr. Perricone to help maintain firmness and tone even during weight loss—are available at:
- N.V. Perricone, M.D., Ltd. at 888-823-7837 or www.nvperriconemd.com
- N.V. Perricone, M.D., Ltd. Flagship Store at 791 Madison Avenue (at 67th St.), New York, NY
- Nordstrom
- Sephora

- ♦ Saks Fifth Avenue
- ♦ Neiman Marcus
- ♦ Henri Bendel
- ♦ Clyde's on Madison (926 Madison Ave. at 74th St., New York, NY)
- ♦ Bloomingdale's
- ♦ Belk's
- ♦ Parisian

EXERCISE

Outstanding information on the benefits and types of exercise, including drawings:
- ♦ President's Council on Physical Fitness (PCPFS). www.fitness.org.
- ♦ The National Institute of Aging. www.niapublications.org.

NUTRITION AND HEALTH INFORMATION

Cancer-preventing Foods
- ♦ The American Institute for Cancer Research. www.aicr.org.

Life Extension Foundation
- ♦ Current scientific news and information on food and nutritional supplements, including the latest on the weight-loss benefits of sesame seeds. An outstanding website! www.lef.org.

Fats of Life and PUFA Newsletter
- ♦ An excellent website and e-mail newsletter concerning essential fatty acids at www.fatsoflife.com.

Food and Nutrition Information Center (USDA)
- ♦ www.nal.usda.gov/fnic/

Outstanding Health and Nutrition Information

♦ WholeHealthMD.com is American WholeHealth Networks' award-winning Complementary and Alternative Medicine (CAM) education website. www.wholehealthmd.com.

Glycemic Index (University of Sydney)

♦ General information on the glycemic index and a searchable foods database at www.glycemicindex.com.

The European Food Information Council

♦ EUFIC is a nonprofit organization that provides science-based information on food and food-related topics to the media, health and nutrition professionals, educators, and opinion leaders. www.eufic.org.

Mercola.com

♦ Information and iconoclastic views from Joseph Mercola, M.D., concerning conventional and alternative medicine and the health implications of various foods and supplements (vitamins, minerals, fatty acids, nutraceuticals, phytoceuticals). www.mercola.com.

National Institutes of Health (NIH)

♦ Links to all NIH centers at www.nih.gov/icd/

Nutrition Source at Harvard School of Public Health

♦ www.hsph.harvard.edu/nutritionsource/index.html

Seafood Safety

♦ Environmental Working Group at www.ewg.org/issues/mercury/2050314/index..php (Mercury issues) and at www.ewg.org/reports/farmedPCBs/part2.php (farmed salmon issues)
♦ Oceans Alive at www.oceansalive.org/eat.cfm?subnav=healthalerts
♦ U.S. Food and Drug Administration Center for Food Safety at www.cfsan.fda.gov/~frf/sea-mehg.html

- ◆ U.S. Environmental Protection Agency (EPA) at www.epa.gov/ost/fish and www.epa.gov/mercury
- ◆ Vital Choice Seafood at www.vitalchoice.com/purity.cfm and www.vitalchoice.com/newsletter_index2.cfm

Soy foods

- ◆ Indiana Soybean Development Council (Stevens & Associates) at www.soyfoods.com
- ◆ Weston A. Price Foundation soy critiques at www.westonaprice.org/soy/index.html and www.westonaprice.org/mythstruths/mtsoy.html

Sweeteners (Noncaloric, Nonglycemic)

- ◆ www.holisticmed.com/sweet
- ◆ Stevia at www.stevia.net
- ◆ Luo Han Kao at www.longjiangriver.com
- ◆ Agave at www.blueagavenectar.com

World's Healthiest Foods (George Mateljan Foundation)

- ◆ Detailed information on healthful whole foods (e.g., fruits, vegetables, nuts, seeds, beans, grains, herbs, spices), including many recipes at www.whfoods.com.

Wheat and Gluten Allergies

- ◆ www.celiac.com

RECIPES

For the recipes featured in the daily meal plan, consult *The Perricone Weight-Loss Diet*, www.amazon.com and at book stores nationwide. For flavorful, healthful recipes, as featured in *The Perricone Weight-Loss Diet*, we recommend

- ◆ *Stop the Clock! Cooking* by Cheryl Forberg, R.D., www.amazon.com